THE
Gastric
Sleeve
BARIATRIC COOKBOOK

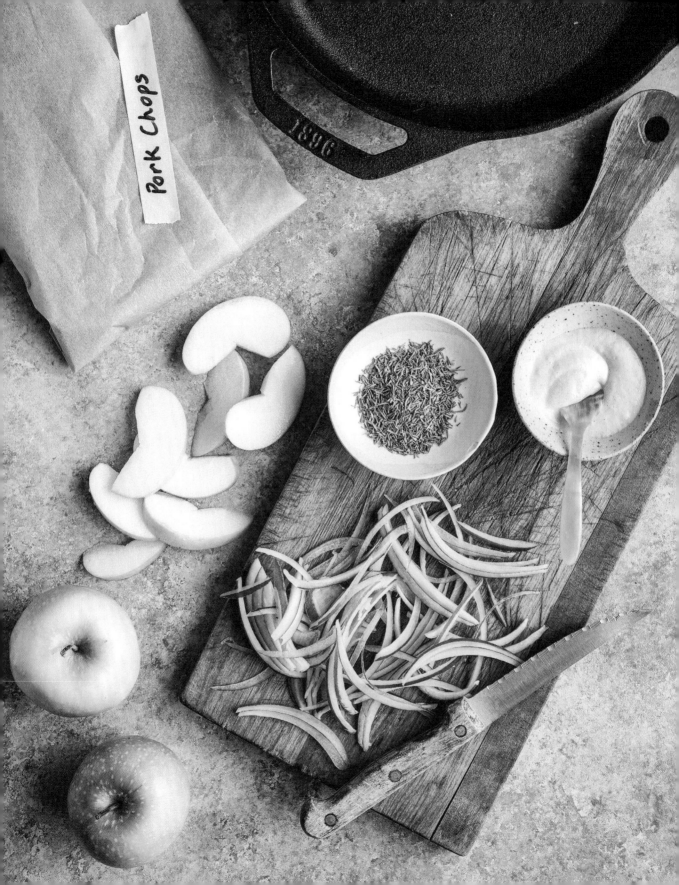

THE
Gastric Sleeve

BARIATRIC COOKBOOK

Easy Meal Plans and Recipes to Eat Well & Keep the Weight Off

SARAH KENT MS, RDN, CSOWM, CD

PHOTOGRAPHY BY HÉLÈNE DUJARDIN

ROCKRIDGE
PRESS

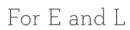

For E and L

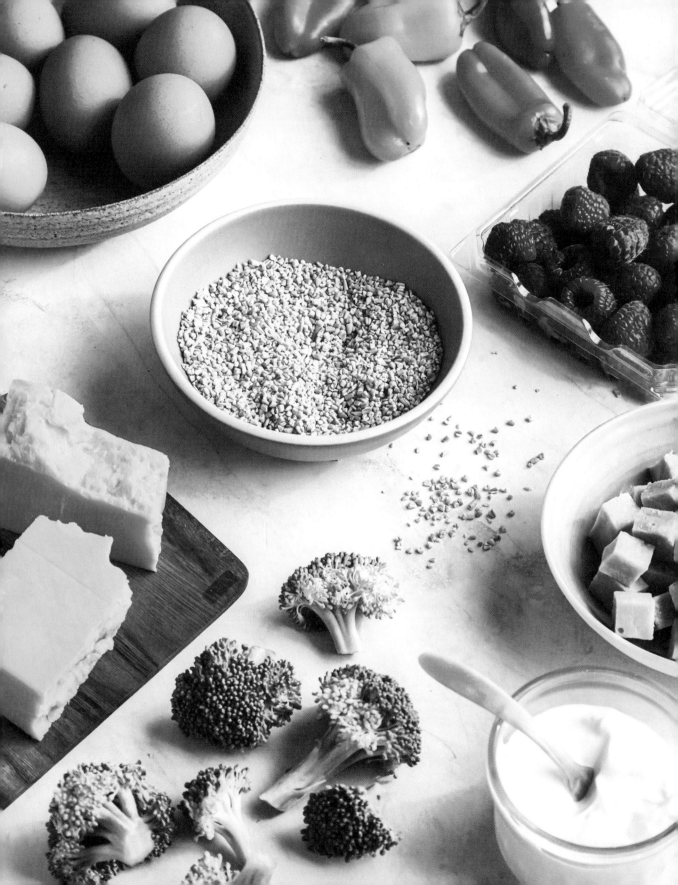

Contents

Introduction

Over the last five years, the number of people in the United States who have undergone the sleeve gastrectomy has more than tripled. The sleeve, sleeve gastrectomy, or vertical sleeve gastrectomy (VSG) has grown to become the most popular type of bariatric surgery, overtaking the Roux-en-Y gastric bypass and adjustable gastric band by a landslide. Bariatric surgery is the most effective procedure in achieving and maintaining significant weight loss when all others have failed. Bariatric surgery can serve as a tool for people who have suffered a lifetime of obesity, people who have uncontrolled health conditions related to obesity that limit their ability to live their lives to the fullest, and people who need to achieve a significant amount of weight loss in a reasonably short amount of time. Whether it's a sleeve gastrectomy or any other type of bariatric surgery, this tool can be life changing. The big key to post-op success is a lifelong commitment to follow specific nutritional guidelines. These strategies will help you achieve success both physically and mentally—and most important, get you healthier and not just thinner.

When you type "bariatric surgery diet" into Google, you get more than 350,000 hits. With this kind of information overload, it's no wonder a person might feel confused about what to eat after weight-loss surgery. I wrote my first cookbook, *Fresh Start Bariatric Cookbook: Healthy Recipes to Enjoy Favorite Foods After Weight-Loss Surgery*, to give people simple guidelines for what to eat and what to avoid after weight-loss surgery. Since it was published, I recognized that people who have been sleeved or are planning to have the sleeve gastrectomy procedure are especially eager for nutritional info that's specific to their needs. Thus this new cookbook, which also includes meal plans for the first few weeks after surgery.

If you've had the VSG, this cookbook will make sure you never have to wonder what to eat, when to eat, or how much to eat. This book is meant to be more than just a resource for recipes. It's a guide for eating after surgery from day 1 until day 10,001. I understand that eating is much more than the food we use to fuel our bodies. There is a relevant emotional component that often accompanies eating, and this book approaches nutrition with both the emotional and nutritional aspects in mind to help people achieve initial and long-term success.

Finally, I want to offer official *congratulations*. You've done it! You've decided to walk away from the latest fad diet, the most recent eating trend, the current weight-loss craze, and you've decided to achieve a healthier lifestyle once and for all. You have taken your need to lose weight seriously and asked for help. You know you can do this, but you also know that you need to pull out the best tool in the toolbox to build your new life. You're tired of yo-yo dieting and you're ready to achieve weight loss permanently. And the best part is, you deserve it. You deserve to feel more energized, to feel lighter, and to go about even the most simple activities in your life with more ease. Most important, you deserve to be healthier. Whether it's breathing easier, leaving some medications behind, or achieving improved test results from your doctor's office—you deserve to experience the perks of a healthier body and mind. Now, let's get to it! Simple guidelines for eating after VSG come first, followed by a book packed with delicious recipes that will satisfy your taste buds and fuel your body. *Bon appétit!*

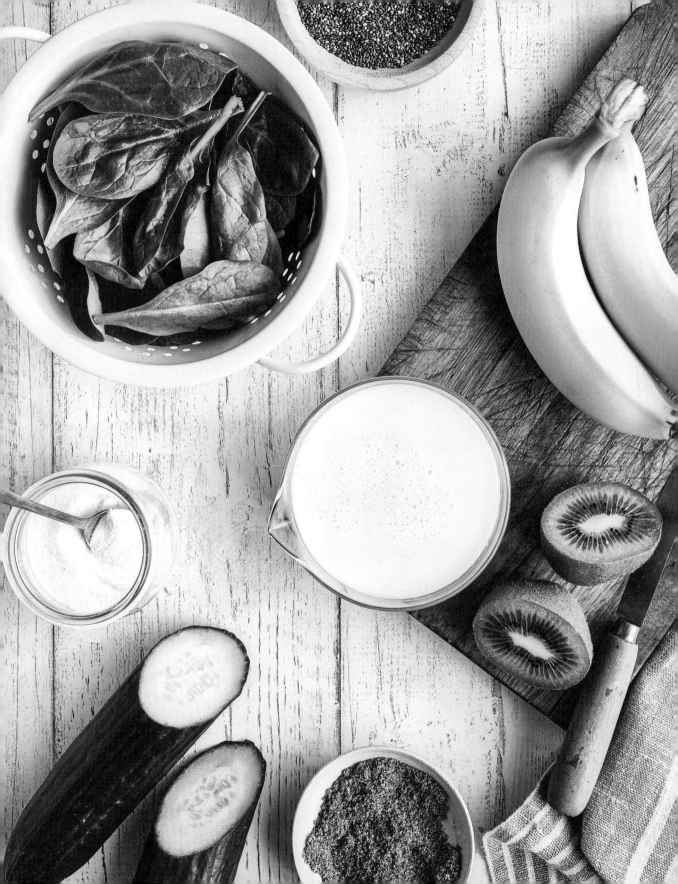

CHAPTER ONE

Welcome to the Sleeve Club

We often crave to be part of a group, a society, a fellowship—well, welcome to the VSG Club! It's a group of people who have had or are planning to have the sleeve gastrectomy. As a registered dietitian who has worked in an academic medical center that is home to a Bariatric Center of Excellence, I know well the struggles people endure long before, and leading up to, their surgery. After deciding to get the procedure and sharing the news with others, some people have overwhelming support from family, friends, and colleagues. Sometimes, however, the responses are negative or misinformed. People may say you're taking the easy way out or that surgery is too drastic and dangerous. These comments need to be thrown out of your mind and replaced with one truth: You are strong. And the unofficial club of people who've had VSG is made up of some of the strongest people in the world, people who have decided—with the validation of medical professionals—to restart and improve their lives once and for all. Congratulations on your strength and bravery.

What Is the Vertical Sleeve Gastrectomy?

As you probably know, there are four main bariatric surgery procedures performed in the United States: The Roux-en-Y gastric bypass, the vertical sleeve gastrectomy (VSG), the adjustable gastric band, and the biliopancreatic diversion with duodenal switch (BPD/DS). Since 2013, the VSG has overtaken the Roux-en-Y gastric bypass as the most common bariatric operation performed in the United States.

The VSG as a unique weight-loss surgery was originally the first part of a two-part bariatric surgery. Some surgeons performed the BPD/DS or gastric bypass as two sequential operations to cut down the risks associated with having one lengthy procedure. First, patients would have a portion of their stomach removed in an initial, shorter, less risky operation—basically a sleeve gastrectomy. Then at a later date, patients returned for the second part of the operation. Weight loss was so successful after the first part of the operation that some patients never returned to complete the second part of the procedure. Thus the VSG was determined to be a successful weight-loss operation with fewer risks than the other procedures and with similar results.

Patients and providers alike love the sleeve gastrectomy. The procedure has gained overwhelming popularity as a single weight-loss operation. During this surgery, the surgeon will remove three-fourths of the original stomach. The banana-shaped stomach left behind is small, so it restricts the amount of food a person can eat at any one time. There are no devices implanted during this operation. No revisions are made to any other part of the person's intestinal tract, which minimizes the risk of long-term nutrient deficiencies. Additionally, the sleeve produces great results when it comes to improving comorbid conditions, such as diabetes and cardiovascular disease. Let's discuss more about why people often choose the sleeve over other types of weight-loss surgeries.

Why Get Sleeved?

Making the choice to have the sleeve gastrectomy over other types of bariatric surgery comes with many advantages. Here are a few reasons why people choose to get sleeved.

1 **Built-in portion control.**
 With about only 15 to 25 percent of your stomach left after surgery, you are limited in the amount of food you can eat at any one time. You can still enjoy a variety of foods with a progression in food texture consistency post-op, but your

stomach will give strong signals to let you know when you are full and trigger you to stop eating.

2 **Fewer hunger pangs.**
With the removal of the majority of the stomach comes a decrease in the hunger hormone ghrelin. Feeling less hunger supports decreased food intake.

3 **Weight loss of more than half your excess body weight.**
Excessive body weight is defined as any pounds above your calculated ideal body weight for your height. Research reported in the *American Society for Metabolic and Bariatric Surgery Integrated Health Nutritional Guidelines for the Surgical Weight Loss Patient* shows that people are able to maintain weight loss of more than 55 percent of their excess body weight five years or longer after surgery. For a person who is 150 pounds over their ideal weight, that means keeping off at least 80 pounds for the long term.

4 **Enjoy sweets without dumping syndrome.**
Most people have a hard time with the concept of committing to giving up birthday cake or special-occasion ice cream for the rest of their life after weight-loss surgery. *Dumping syndrome* is a condition that can occur in people who have had the gastric bypass or BPD/DS surgery after eating foods high in sugar and, in some cases, eating too many carbohydrates at one time. Symptoms occur shortly after consuming the food in question and include some combination of feeling shaky, light-headed, sweaty, or dizzy; increased heart rate; a drop in blood sugar levels (reactive hypoglycemia); abdominal cramping; and diarrhea. Although large quantities of sweets could still cause dumping-like symptoms after a VSG, it's very uncommon and not as severe as after weight-loss surgeries that involve modifying the small intestine.

5 **Less time in the operating room.**
Any operation performed under general anesthesia includes risks and the potential for complications. These risks can multiply with the amount of time the operation takes to be completed. Although the VSG is a lengthier procedure than the adjustable band, it is a shorter and simpler procedure than the gastric bypass and the BPD/DS.

Starting Over with Food

A full team of medical professionals, including, at minimum, a surgeon, a registered dietitian, and a psychologist, will help you more fully understand your surgery as well as how to prepare for it physically, mentally, and nutritionally. But in the days, weeks, and years after surgery, success will come down to your ability to truly and lastingly start over with food. Half of this restart involves self-education about nutrition (see page 10) and the other half involves self-management, which can be the hardest part. On the next few pages, I discuss the top challenges people face after surgery.

IF YOU'RE CONSIDERING GASTRIC BYPASS

The main difference between the gastric bypass and VSG is the second step of the gastric bypass procedure that involves rerouting part of the small intestinal tract. During the gastric bypass procedure, a small pouch is created from the larger stomach and part of the small intestinal tract is divided and connected to the new stomach. As a result, the lower part of the stomach and the top portion of the small intestinal tract are "bypassed" during the digestion of food.

Compared with the sleeve gastrectomy, the gastric bypass produces slightly greater weight loss in the short term and has slightly better resolution rates of type 2 diabetes. After gastric bypass, dumping syndrome can occur when patients eat sweets. Dumping syndrome is often a helpful deterrent from eating sweets for people who struggle with limiting calorie intake from sugary foods.

One other difference between the gastric bypass and sleeve gastrectomy is that after the operation, the gastric bypass will immediately resolve any symptoms of gastroesophageal reflux disease, or GERD. After a VSG, reflux may actually become worse immediately after the operation, but often improves with time. It's very important to discuss the nature of your own habits and health history in detail with your surgeon and medical team to determine which surgery really is best for you for the long term.

When it comes to post-op nutrition, the guidelines for the gastric bypass and VSG are very similar. You can still prepare all of this book's recipes without concern for texture or portion if you opt for the bypass.

Embracing Eating Without Fear

Having bariatric surgery means you agree to learn how to eat all over again. Starting with only liquids, you will gradually progress to a balanced diet of nearly all the foods you could eat before surgery. You might be fearful of knowing exactly what is safe to eat and not really want to eat again because of this fear. Additionally you might be fearful of falling into old eating habits and undoing the benefits of the surgery. In order to embrace eating without fear, focus on what you *can* eat instead of what you *can't* eat.

▶ **Stick to the basic principles of the bariatric diet and choose to eat foods you know you can have.** It's going to take months for you to get completely confident with the dos and don'ts of the bariatric diet, so give yourself time and don't experiment right away. If you stick to the rules for the first several weeks, you won't get sick. Period. After that, listen to the signals from your body.

▶ **Be mindful and make every effort to stop eating at the first sign of fullness.** Tap into the natural signals your body will give you and resist eating another bite when you feel full. You don't have to live in fear; your body will tell you when to stop.

▶ **Commit to yourself.** This time really is different. You might be afraid of going back to the "old you" just like other times you have dieted in the past. But now you have the help of this beneficial surgery, which gives you a great head start. Now you're not simply starting a diet, you're beginning an entire lifestyle change: a permanent lifestyle change with no turning back.

▶ **Recognize that support is paramount.** Rely on your medical professionals at a minimum, and hopefully at least a few friends, family, or colleagues. Turn to the people you trust for encouragement when you're feeling afraid. If you feel like you have no one who will support you, check again. There is *someone*—a bariatric support group, a health coach, a psychologist, a pastor, a colleague. Connect with that person who can help cheer you on through the bumps in the road. Living in fear disables you mentally and physically. Be confident that you can be successful post-op and be mindful each day of the choices you make.

Controlling Urges

We all have urges. Whether it's an impulse purchase at the mall, a second helping of dessert, or a wasted day watching Netflix and missing your workout—there are plenty of opportunities to give in to impulse and fall off track from your healthy lifestyle. Controlling urges involves two parts.

1 **Develop mindfulness.** Being aware of your thoughts, feelings, and actions in the present moment can help you suppress impulses.

2 **Don't give in to cravings.** For some people, giving in to an urge means flipping a switch, turning something back into the "on" position that may have been suppressed. How many times does eating one chip turn into half a bag, drinking one glass of wine turn into half a bottle, or eating one Oreo turn into the entire sleeve? For many bariatric patients, giving in to an urge, compulsion, or impulse may lead to a binge-type of behavior. Practice mindfulness and ask yourself if this is what your body really needs in the moment. Sometimes the answer is "yes," it is what you need. But stop yourself and ask twice before giving in to a small urge, as it often leads to a domino effect of self-harming behaviors.

Demonstrating Self-Compassion

How we feel about ourselves and how we treat ourselves following both good and bad behaviors directly affects our happiness. It can also influence our ability to stick with long-term behavior changes following surgery. Dr. Kristin Neff defines self-compassion as comprising three parts—self-kindness, mindfulness, and common humanity.

▶ **All patients make mistakes after surgery.** It's whether we respond with self-compassion or self-criticism that determines how resilient we are after a period of sliding back into old habits. We are all human and we have our imperfections. Embrace your good qualities and embrace your struggles, too.

▶ **Try to leverage your strengths to use them to overcome barriers in other areas.** Self-denigration will only move you farther away from your goals. When you have a few bad days, understand that your mind may have needed a break.

▶ **Try to move on without focusing too much on past mistakes, and look forward to your continued success.**

Appreciating Natural Sweetness

We live in a culture where our threshold for sweetness is getting higher and higher. Desserts are getting more sugary and sweet drinks are getting sweeter. Breaking the habit of eating sweets can be especially difficult for anyone trying to lose weight because sugar is addicting. Eating sugary foods turns on pleasure centers in your brain, making you want to go back for more. If this is something you have been struggling with, bariatric surgery gives you an opportunity to press the reset button. You get a redo on your eating patterns and the chance to get some major help in kicking old habits to the curb.

Focus on eating naturally sweet foods to balance your need to satisfy all taste buds. Include grains such as barley or quinoa, which have a sweet and nutty flavor and are still loaded with lots of nutrients. Instead of sugary desserts, cap off your meal with something naturally sweet like fresh berries or refreshing citrus fruits. Even using 100 percent cocoa powder in protein shakes or other baked goods can curb your chocolate craving without the extra sugar and fat from typical milk chocolate candies. Appreciating the natural sweetness in foods can help push your sugar addiction aside!

MANAGING WEIGHT-LOSS EXPECTATIONS

Weight loss is not a perfect science. Even in a controlled weight-loss research study, there still is some variance on the amount of weight individuals lose. It's frustrating when you give something 110 percent effort and the results aren't what you want. In order to manage your expectations about weight loss post-op, don't put undue pressure on yourself to lose weight faster than what is realistic. Know yourself. Other people may lose weight faster or slower than you do. The factors that go into weight loss are multifaceted and some are out of your control. Did you know that weight loss might even be affected by the amount of sleep you get? In addition to food intake, exercise, muscle mass, stress, starting body weight, height, gender, age, and even more factors all play a part in the amount of weight you will lose. Be diligent, yet patient, and don't compare yourself to others. Your weight-loss journey is unique; it's okay and expected that you will be frustrated at times. Just know that with continued hard work you will achieve long-term success.

Enjoying Food Again

During the first few days post-op, when you're consuming mostly liquids, it's hard to imagine you'll ever find delight in eating food again. Initially, eating may become a chore, something done out of necessity. Questions may start to flutter: Will I look forward to eating again? Will I ever be able to eat the foods I used to love?

Keep in mind that right after surgery, your body rapidly undergoes physical and hormonal changes—all of which suppress your urge to eat and the amount you are able to eat. Most of your initial rapid weight loss is a product of the combination of these changes. Be patient. As time progresses you will be interested in and able to eat a slightly larger volume of food and tolerate more variety of foods.

I know this may sound crazy, but some people who really craved pizza and ice cream before surgery may no longer have a desire for those types of foods. As you transition to eating a diet full of nutritious foods and leave behind high-calorie foods, you'll find that your body begins to crave the healthier foods more. And that's the perfect time to try some of your favorite old recipes—with a healthier twist.

Food is nourishment for your body; it's a necessity to eat every single day. But mealtime is so much more than just what we put in our bodies. With a little bit of time, patience, and a willingness to experiment, enjoying nutritious foods is truly possible after surgery.

The Sweet Stuff

Unlike with the gastric bypass or BPD/DS, dumping syndrome is not really a risk with VSG. This means desserts—in the proper portions—are not off the table after surgery. Patients often have concerns after surgery about feeling "normal" while having to be on a special diet. Going to restaurants, family gatherings, and parties can be uncomfortable if you have to explain why you can't even have a bite of dessert because you would be in the bathroom all night. Choosing the sleeve offers more flexibility around some of the social eating you do, so you'll have to offer fewer explanations.

I still strongly advise you to be careful not to overindulge, and here are a few basic tips to help.

- ▸ Save the sweet stuff for special occasions.

- ▸ Don't keep temping desserts in your home.

- ▸ Don't keep a candy dish on your desk.

- ▸ Always use portion-controlled desserts—individual servings versus the big bag.

Research has shown that if you sit down with the entire bag of cookies you're going to eat much more than if you sit down with one individual serving in a small dish. Even if you go back for seconds, always start with a small single serving—you will eat less overall. Bottom line: If you choose, sweets can still be an option in your post-op diet. It's up to you how to include them to keep calories in check.

Meal Planning

Just like brushing your teeth, wearing your seat belt, or even getting dressed in the morning, meal planning should be an integrated part of your new lifestyle. Mapping out your meals for the week doesn't have to mean tediously detailing every ingredient; it means that you know about 75 percent of the foods you will be eating over the next few days. You know you have the ingredients on hand and which staples you've stocked for the days when you aren't preparing a meal from scratch.

Meal planning is especially important in the first few months post-op to make sure you get enough protein. Plan your meals centered on the protein first and then next work on adding in fruits and vegetables. Introduce grains and other foods last. When you plan your meals ahead of time, you know you'll always have something healthy and properly portioned that you can eat. It takes the stress out of the day-to-day routine, prevents you from getting overly hungry, and reduces the temptation to order or buy something unhealthy. Remember that you can often cook a meal once and eat it twice (or more!). Freeze leftovers for later. Make your own "frozen dinners" by portioning food into reusable containers and freezing them. Keep a running list on a notepad of what's in your freezer—when you made it and where you put it—so nothing gets lost. Anything with a sauce tends to freeze well and stay moist when reheated. After flavors continue to meld, your meal may be even tastier as a leftover! The first couple of months post-op can be especially hard, so this book includes meal plans in the next chapter for the first eight weeks to show you how to use this book's recipes for a complete post-op eating program.

VSG Nutritional Know-How

By the time most people undergo bariatric surgery, they are quite familiar with common weight-loss diets. You're likely well familiar with the nutritional benefits and restrictions of various diets, from Weight Watchers to the Mediterranean diet, from Atkins to the DASH diet. Fortunately, what you've already learned about following diets in the past will serve as a foundation for learning how to eat after bariatric surgery. You don't need to be a nutrition expert to understand and follow a bariatric eating plan. Let's review the principles for eating after surgery, which are represented throughout the recipes in this cookbook.

Liquids

Staying hydrated after surgery is the first and most important rule. Drinking enough liquids will not only increase your energy, but it will also help significantly with your weight loss. Additionally, dehydration is the most common complication post-op, and one that can easily be prevented. It can be challenging at first, partly because you cannot drink with meals or 30 minutes before or after eating. Be proactive and always carry a beverage with you. Focus on drinking small amounts throughout the morning and afternoon to prevent trying to catch up later—and remember that your smaller stomach will prohibit you from chugging large amounts of fluid at one time.

What to Drink: water, milk, soy milk, protein shakes, decaffeinated tea or coffee (without added cream or sugar), and any other noncarbonated and sugar-free beverages (sweetened with sugar substitutes is okay)

Amount per Day: 64 to 100 ounces—progressing in volume throughout your post-op diet stages

What to Limit or Avoid: juices, caffeinated beverages (including soda, coffee, tea, and energy drinks), carbonated waters, alcohol, lemonade, sweetened tea, sports drinks, and any sugar-sweetened beverages

Protein

It's all about protein, which is the most important macronutrient to take in post-op. Protein is the building block of muscle and tissue. It's crucial to eat adequate protein while following a very low-calorie diet. When you eat enough protein, you will feel energized, lose more fat while preserving muscle, and experience longer post-meal satisfaction. Protein is digested more slowly than carbohydrates and contains fewer calories than fats. Initially post-op, it will seem like you are taking in only water and protein-rich foods. As you progress, you will slowly add more mixed meals into your diet. This cookbook is essential to give you a variety of ideas for eating adequate protein for the long haul so meals don't become boring. Turn to page 16 for a table of protein-rich foods, along with portion sizes and protein grams for each. Eating protein at every meal for a lifetime is essential to not only lose weight and heal initially, but also to maintain weight loss for the long term.

What to Eat: eggs, poultry (chicken and turkey without skin, lean nitrate-free chicken or turkey sausage, ground chicken and turkey breast), all fish and seafood, low-fat or nonfat dairy products (low-fat Greek yogurt, 1% or nonfat cottage cheese, 1% or nonfat milk and cheese), lean beef (if tolerated) beginning three months post-op (sirloin, loin, round roast or steak, and lean or supreme lean ground beef), lean pork (if tolerated) beginning three months post-op (tenderloin, top loin chop, and ham with visible fat removed), and vegetarian protein sources (beans, nuts, lentils, and seeds)

Amount per Day: 60 to 100 grams (Note: Specific recommendations are based on ideal body weight and post-op diet stage.)

What to Limit or Avoid: high-fat dairy products (cream and whole milk), high-fat cuts of beef or pork (pork sausage, bacon, bologna, salami, pork ribs, and ground beef), and skin-on poultry

Carbohydrates

A quick source of energy for your body, including your brain, carbohydrates are important for many metabolic functions. During the initial post-op diet, you will take in few to no carbs. Your body will function normally by obtaining energy from metabolizing fat stores and using protein from the foods you do eat. Carbohydrates can be found in two varieties: simple or complex. Simple carbohydrates are digested quickly and easily turn into sugar in our blood, giving us a quick energy rush and subsequent crash. Simple carbs include foods made with white refined flour, candies, soda, juice drinks, and many processed foods. Complex carbohydrates are digested more slowly and are rich in fiber, vitamins, and minerals. They include 100% whole-grain foods, fruits, and vegetables. Focus on limiting simple carbs and eating more complex carbs.

What to Eat: fresh fruits, vegetables, sweet potatoes or white potatoes with skin, oatmeal, 100 percent whole-grain bread products (toasted is better tolerated than doughy fresh), brown or wild rice or 100 percent whole-wheat pasta (if tolerated), and barley and ancient grains (quinoa, spelt, farrow, millet)

Amount per Day: very small amounts initially; after the first year and long-term, aim for 35 to 45 percent total calories from carbohydrates

What to Limit or Avoid: any white refined grain products (white bread, white pasta, and crackers), cookies, candies, cakes, pastries, juices (including fruit juice), soda, and chips

Fats

Dietary fats are important to absorb the essential fat-soluble vitamins—A, D, E, and K. Additionally there are some essential fatty acids (omega-3s and omega-6s) our bodies cannot make and must ingest instead. Fats are the most calorie-dense of all macronutrients at nine calories per gram, so we must always be careful of portion sizes—even in the healthy versions. Be cautious with processed foods labeled as fat free or low fat as they often replace fat with more sugar or sodium to improve the flavor of the food. Dairy products, particularly milk, yogurt, and cottage cheese, should be eaten in low-fat or nonfat form to save on calories and artery-clogging saturated fats. Choose these versions when cooking as often as possible. Note that nonfat or 1% milk does not contain any fewer vitamins, minerals, or grams of protein than whole milk. Choose full-fat foods in the form of vegetable oils, nuts, seeds, avocados, olives, and fatty fish—all of which are heart healthy.

What to Eat: avocado, chia seeds, fatty fish (salmon, mackerel, and tuna), other seafood and shellfish, flaxseed, extra-virgin olive oil, almonds, walnuts, peanuts, and all-natural nut butters

Amount per Day: very limited amounts initially; long term no more than 30 percent of your total calories should be from fats (mostly healthy versions and less than 7 percent from saturated fats)

What to Limit: butter, tropical oils (palm and coconut oil), full-fat dairy, and miscellaneous vegetable oils

What to Avoid: animal fats (fat on meats, lard), fried foods, stick margarines containing trans fats, and foods high in processed saturated fats

Vitamin and Mineral Supplements

Food is the best source of the nutrients for your body after the VSG. Because of the restricted amount of food they are able to eat, however, all bariatric surgery patients need to take vitamin and mineral supplements post-op. Follow the recommendations from your bariatric surgery team for specific details. Beyond those specifics, here are some general recommendations.

Take your vitamins as close to mealtime as possible. Some vitamins are best absorbed when accompanied by food. It's okay to break the rule of "no liquids with meals" to take just a few sips to get down your pills if you are taking a capsule or tablet version.

Avoid using gummy vitamins post-op. Most versions are high in sugar, are high in calories, and do not meet the 100 to 200 percent recommended daily allowance for all vitamins and minerals. If you find a version that meets your nutritional needs, verify it first with your medical team to make sure it's approved for you.

Look for supplements with the USP verified symbol. Since herbal supplements and vitamins are not regulated by the FDA, this symbol lets you to know you are getting a high-quality brand. You may choose to purchase specialty vitamins from companies like Bariatric Advantage or Celebrate vitamins, which are targeted to weight-loss surgery patients. Keep in mind that specialty supplements are expensive and they aren't necessary if you choose the proper over-the-counter equivalents. However, you might choose these brands to take the guesswork out of making sure you are getting the right formula of supplements.

What follows is a list of vitamin supplements that may be recommended for you to take. Always follow the advice of your medical team.

▸ **Multivitamin with minerals, in chewable or liquid form (at least for the first 6 months).** Make sure the vitamins and minerals supply 200 percent of the daily recommended value, which often requires two tablets per day in a split dose.

▸ **Vitamin D is advised for most everyone, since nearly all who qualify for the surgery tend to be deficient in it.** A commonly recommended dosage is 3,000 IU per day and often more depending on baseline levels.

▸ **Calcium is recommended for most all patients post-op because of the importance of bone health.** Aim for 1,200 to 1,500 mg per day in two or three divided doses.

▸ **Iron may be recommended based on your levels.** Iron is important for red blood cells, which carry oxygen throughout your body. It is not standard to universally recommend supplemental iron after a sleeve gastrectomy, but depending on your levels you may require additional iron.

▶ **Vitamin B$_{12}$ absorption may be impaired after the VSG.** This vitamin is important for preventing anemia and for normal nerve function. Look at your routine post-op lab results to see if you need additional B$_{12}$ supplementation. It's often administered through an injection or a daily oral supplement of 1,000 mcg per day.

Bottom line: Because of the nature of the VSG, taking certain vitamin and mineral supplements is a commitment for life. I have seen deficiencies appear several years down the road when people reach their goal weight and stop taking their supplements. Make sure to follow up regularly with your medical team to have your blood levels of these important nutrients tested.

TYPE 2 DIABETES AND BARIATRIC SURGERY

Weight-loss surgery shows great promise for resolving type 2 diabetes. Remarkably, resolution of diabetes appears to be independent of weight loss. Many people leave the hospital with normal blood sugar control and without any medication. The "cure" of type 2 diabetes alone is reason enough for many people to undergo the operation. Several research studies indicate that gastric bypass is the best operation for overcoming diabetes, but we're learning it's not so black and white. According to the American Society for Metabolic and Bariatric Surgery, 60 percent of patients with diabetes experience remission of type 2 diabetes after the sleeve gastrectomy. After the gastric bypass, results are up to about 80 percent. It appears that the likelihood for remission may also be linked to how many years a person has had diabetes and their degree of insulin resistance. In most patients, there is a huge improvement in disease management even in absence of complete remission. The surgery works in two major ways to improve blood sugar control. The drastic initial improvement after surgery is related to gut hormones and improved utilization of the insulin your body produces. Long term, the weight loss, diet changes, and improved physical activity support blood sugar control.

The Bariatric Kitchen

Your kitchen is your workshop after surgery. Fortunately, you don't need a complete kitchen makeover to eat well. You just need a few important staples and pieces of equipment to prepare fast, delicious meals and ensure long-term weight-loss success. Here's a table of which foods to get rid of and the healthier foods that should replace them.

Toss It	Stock Up
Vegetable oil	Extra-virgin olive oil
All-purpose flour	Whole-wheat pastry flour
Sour cream	Low-fat plain Greek yogurt, hummus
Processed cheeses and cheese spreads	Natural cheeses (mozzarella, Cheddar, feta, etc.), cottage cheese
Canned premade soups	Canned or dried beans for making homemade soups, low-sodium broth
Hot dogs, bacon	100 percent natural nitrate-free chicken or nitrate-free turkey sausage
Instant oatmeal packets	100 percent old-fashioned rolled oats or steel-cut oats, unsweetened
Fruit snacks	Fresh fruits, 100 percent natural (unsweetened) applesauce, fruit cups in water or drained from natural juice, frozen fruit
Salami, bologna, pastrami	Nitrate-free deli-sliced turkey, chicken, ham, lean roast beef
Juice	Fresh lemons and limes sliced for water, herbal tea
Potato chips and pretzels	Dehydrated vegetables/snap peas (Snapea Crisps or Lentil Snaps), kale chips
Flavored regular yogurt	Plain yogurt, lower-sugar Greek yogurt
Canned high-fat meats or sausages	Canned chicken breast; packets or cans of tuna, salmon, crab, shrimp
Pasta	Fresh spaghetti squash and spiralized zucchini
Creamy processed salad dressings	Flavored vinegars and extra-virgin olive oil, yogurt-based dressings

Protein-Rich Foods

Counting grams of protein can help you make sure you are getting what you need. You can use an app on your smartphone, such as MyFitnessPal, to keep track electronically, or use the following chart to keep track by hand.

Protein Source	Portion Size	Protein (grams)*
Poultry, beef, pork, fish	2 ounces	14 grams (7 grams per ounce)
Shrimp, scallops	3 ounces (about 15 large)	18 grams
Lunch meat (nitrate-free turkey, chicken, ham, or roast beef)	2 ounces (4 to 6 thin slices)	10 grams
Eggs	1 large	6 to 7 grams
Egg whites	2 large	8 grams
Cottage or ricotta cheese (fat free, 1% to 2% fat)	½ cup	14 grams
Natural cheese (Cheddar, Colby, mozzarella, Swiss, etc.)	1 ounce or 1 slice	7 grams
Greek yogurt (nonfat, low fat)	6 ounces (¾ cup)	10 to 15 grams
Yogurt (nonfat, low fat)	6 ounces (¾ cup)	5 grams
Lentils	½ cup cooked	9 grams
Beans	½ cup cooked	5 to 9 grams

Individual protein content may vary; always check the nutrition facts label

Foods to Avoid After Surgery

The long-term post-op goal is to live a normal life, eating most foods in moderation. A big fear patients have is abdominal discomfort or vomiting after surgery. During the first three months after surgery, some foods should be avoided completely to prevent this scenario from occurring, but many foods can be slowly added over time as your body adjusts to its "new" stomach.

Liquids	Carbonated beverages, alcohol, caffeinated beverages, fruit juices, any sugary beverages
Proteins	Dry, tough meat and poultry, any breaded or deep-fried proteins
Carbohydrates	Rice, pasta, doughy bread products (untoasted breads), dried fruits, skin-on fruit, fresh pineapple, popcorn, dry fibrous cereals, such as granola and bran cereal
Fats	Raw nuts/seeds, fried foods, greasy foods (skin-on poultry, fat-on meat), peanut and other nut butters (sticky)
Other Foods	Asparagus stalks, raw celery, coconut, sugar-sweetened sauces/condiments, cookies, candy

Food Texture Week by Week

Diet progression should be guided by your individual bariatric team; however, here is a list of general guidelines. Most people are eating foods with general consistency within six to eight weeks post-op.

Post-Operative Timeline	Diet Type
Days 1 to 2	Clear liquid diet
Weeks 1 to 2	(FL) Full liquid diet
Week 3	(P) Pureed foods
Weeks 4 to 6	(S) Soft foods
Weeks 7 or 8+	(G) Advance to general foods

Equipment

You will find that the majority of the recipes in this book require very little more than a cutting board, sauté pan, and a good knife! Here are a few must-have kitchen tools to help you prepare some of the recipes in this cookbook. You can find most of them at major department stores for a reasonable price.

Immersion or hand blender For pureeing soups, chilies, sauces, or other dishes while still on the stove

Spiralizer For making zucchini noodles (to replace pasta); try the small handheld versions

Muffin tin Great for portion control; have the regular and mini versions on hand for different options

Blender or food processor (dishwasher safe) For pureeing small portions of foods for yourself or to make a single-serving shake

Slow cooker Five-quart size is sufficient for the recipes in this book; you may opt for smaller or larger versions

Vegetable peeler For removing tough skins from fruits and vegetables that aren't tolerated during the first few months post-op

Air fryer Although not necessary to make any recipes in this book, the air fryer is all the rage as a substitute for deep-frying foods. It's an option. Use extra-virgin olive oil spray to make crispy "fried" veggies without all the fat from typical fried foods.

THE ROLE OF FRUIT

Sugar gets a lot of attention these days because of the negative side effects it can have on a person's health and waistline. Unfortunately, sugars get lumped into one big category and sometimes good sugars, like the kind in fruit, also get a bad rap. In the upcoming years, nutrition facts labels will start listing added sugars versus naturally occurring sugars. Whole fruits will have a big zero in the added sugars section. In addition to beneficial phytochemicals, fruit also contains loads of fiber, which can delay the absorption of the fruit's natural sugar. Note these cautions regarding fruit intake: Fruit does not have any protein. Eat your protein first; then add other foods like fruit. Fruit is higher in calories and carbohydrates than vegetables. One cup of fresh berries or melon, one small apple, or half a banana all have around 60 calories and 15 grams carbohydrates. Fill up on vegetables, which are mega-packed with nutrients and low in carbohydrates, before fruit. For the long haul, include about two servings of fruit per day and no more than four. Berries are a great choice since they are mega-packed with nutrients. Dried fruit and fruit juices are not recommended as they are high in sugar and calories.

Frequently Asked Questions

After surgery, stay connected with your medical bariatric team and a support group so that you can easily get answers to your questions and concerns from a reliable source—and receive support and encouragement. Here are a few questions that I encountered frequently in my practice.

I've never tried protein powders before. What recommendations do you have?

Taking a walk down the protein and supplement aisle in your grocery store can be overwhelming. There are hundreds of products on the market, each one claiming to be better than the next. You want to set a solid plan of eating food since you are not going to drink protein shakes for the rest of your life. The protein shakes and powders should be a bridge for the first few days and weeks post-op to enable you to eat whole foods. Additionally, protein powders can be used to help you easily take in a dense source of high-quality protein with very few calories. Here are my guidelines for bariatric-friendly protein powders.

▶ **Choose whey protein isolate.** It's easiest for your body to absorb and is dense in essential amino acids. Try the brands biPro or UNJURY. Other high-quality sources include soy protein isolate (vegan) or egg white powder.

▶ **Try an unflavored protein powder.** These are low in calories and the cleanest since they're free from artificial ingredients.

▶ **For flavored protein powders, choose sugar-free.** That's right, look for completely sugar-free varieties that are sweetened with stevia, sucralose (Splenda), or other sugar substitutes. There are hundreds of flavor options from vanilla to butter pecan, which will leave you satisfied for very few calories. Sugar substitutes are FDA-approved, calorie-free, and safe to have after surgery. Be cautious with sugar alcohols (erythritol, mannitol, xylitol, and sorbitol) as they contribute some calories, and consumption can cause unpleasant gastrointestinal side effects.

▶ **Find sample sizes to try before your surgery.** Check on the manufacturer's website for free or discounted offers. That way you'll know what you like and what you don't so you're set up for the first few days post-op.

If I haven't eaten enough protein throughout the day, what can I eat at the end of the day to meet my protein goal?

Go for something quick and easy, such as low-fat cottage cheese or Greek yogurt, hard-boiled eggs, nitrate-free turkey or chicken lunch meat, or low-fat cheese. Milk or a protein shake can also satisfy to meet your protein goal. The key is to focus on hitting your protein goal at least 80 percent of the time. Start the next day with a high-protein breakfast to make up for what you may have missed the day before.

I get full so quickly on the protein in my meals. Will I ever have enough room for fruits and vegetables?

Yes. It seems impossible that eating straight protein foods for weeks and months on end could be considered a healthy lifestyle, but it's only temporary. Your multi-vitamin will cover what you will lack in nutrients during this time. Focus on making it a priority to eat fruits and vegetables as the first foods you include once you are able to branch out past proteins. Vary fruit and vegetable types throughout the week since it's challenging to eat several servings in one day. There are dozens of recipes in this book that give tips for how to sneak fruits and vegetables right into your protein main dishes. Work your way up to five total servings of fruits and veggies per day for the long term.

I keep getting different information about eating carbs. Is it okay to eat bread and pasta after surgery?

There are two different reasons people avoid eating doughy bread products and pasta after surgery. The first is that they are poorly tolerated by your new stomach. During the first few months, the sleeve has a hard time digesting these foods. If you eat them, you may feel overly full quickly and then hungry shortly after, or feel bloated, and/or experience the feeling that something is stuck in your small stomach. These symptoms usually pass after the first few months, but some patients report discomfort from eating these types of foods even in the long term. The second reason people limit carbohydrate intake is to put more focus on eating protein foods for fullness and fruits and vegetables, which are low in calories. It's not bad to eat bread and pasta after surgery if you can tolerate them—it should just be in moderation, with the focus on protein first, then vegetables, then carbohydrates.

I'm really committed to this diet, but my spouse just wants to keep eating junk food all the time. How do I keep on track if I don't have 100 percent support in my household?

It's ideal to enlist the support of loved ones, partners, family, and friends prior to surgery but you can't always wait to make a lifestyle change until everyone you know is equally ready. Here are a few tips for staying on track when the rest of the household might be more resistant.

▶ **Keep your most tempting treats out of the pantry.** Only allow treats on hand that you can resist. Maybe Oreos are your biggest weakness, but the rest of the household couldn't care less if the cookies are Chips Ahoy or Nutter Butters. Don't buy Oreos but allow family favorites that don't tempt you.

▶ **Find an outlet.** Whether it's heading out for a walk, going to bed early, getting lost in a good book, or calling a friend—find an outlet for stress, anxiety, or boredom that isn't eating. Make sure you have an alternative activity for yourself when the potato chips are calling your name.

▶ **Keep simple meals on hand for yourself and the rest of the family.** Make every effort to avoid becoming a short-order cook post-op. Keep some go-to meals on hand so there is always something healthy, quick, and easy around. If possible, choose meals that can easily be modified to meet your needs and others' flavor preferences.

▶ **Ask for what you need.** Not everyone in the household may understand your needs when following the bariatric diet. Practice good communication and make sure you are clear in what you need for support. You can't assume that other people know what your goals are and what you need to reach them.

Am I going to have to follow a special preoperative diet before bariatric surgery?

Weight-loss surgery is an operation on your stomach, but it doesn't change the eating habits ingrained in your brain pre-operatively. With that in mind, I strongly suggest that patients establish as many healthy and positive eating patterns ahead of time with the post-op diet in mind. Getting habits in line before surgery can make things much easier when you are recovering. It's overwhelming to ask yourself to figure out how to count protein grams, give up fast food, stop drinking liquids with meals, and start taking multivitamin supplements all at one time. Whether or not your surgical center requires that you follow a pre-operative diet of some kind is independent of your choice to establish as many of the post-op habits as possible ahead of time. Many bariatric surgery programs and/or insurance companies require some sort of pre-operative weight loss, high-protein diet, or liquid diet during the days, weeks, and sometimes months before surgery. Losing weight in the last week or two before surgery, especially through a low-carbohydrate or liquid diet, may help reduce the size of the liver and decrease belly fat, which could make the operation easier for the surgeon and safer for you.

Just Keep Trying

When you wake up from bariatric surgery, your entire lifestyle will change only if you choose to make it different. Surgery does not stop you from eating fast food. Surgery does not make you get off the couch to exercise. Surgery does not stop you from cozying up with a bag of potato chips at night. Modifying a lifetime of habits to achieve your weight-loss goals can be challenging. Although you will encounter barriers and obstacles, just keep trying. Babies don't learn how to run before they can walk. So just try small things. Maybe you can walk only for 10 minutes without getting tired, but 10 minutes is a start. Maybe you can't give up sweets completely, but you can swap in smaller servings. Maybe you can't give up fast food, but you can get the burger without a side of fries. Small steps make a difference. Set realistic, achievable goals for yourself. You will have weeks when the pounds fall off in double digits and weeks when you can't seem to make the scale budge. Do not give up. Do not lose hope. Just keep trying. Keep a food log again for a couple of days. Try a new

ALCOHOL AFTER VSG

If you enjoyed a few alcoholic beverages before bariatric surgery and you're wondering if this is something you can continue post-op, you should have a good understanding of how your surgery can affect the absorption of alcohol. There is an enzyme in the stomach that helps to partially digest alcohol. Since the majority of the stomach is removed after the VSG, your ability to break down alcohol will be greatly altered. As a result, even a small amount of alcohol intake will be extremely intoxicating. Your smaller body size and decreased food intake will also contribute to alcohol intoxication and dehydration. Also, alcohol is extremely calorie dense. Bariatric surgery does not restrict liquid calories and calories from alcohol can add up very quickly.

Weddings, family gatherings, parties—alcohol can be a big part of socializing, but for many post-op patients, alcohol intake can be a substitute for food as an escape from stress. According to the Obesity Action Coalition, the risk of alcoholism is increased after bariatric surgery because of something called addiction transfer. People trade food for alcohol as an outlet for stress, depression, or anxiety. So think twice before popping the champagne after surgery—consider making yourself the designated driver and go for nonalcoholic beverages instead.

If alcoholism is a concern for you or a loved one, know that your bariatric medical team is there to support you; help is waiting. Alcoholism should not be kept secret and you are not alone. You can also find information on Alcoholics Anonymous in this book's Resources section (page 182). Alcoholics Anonymous can help you determine if you have an addiction transfer problem and help you battle it.

fitness class. Go to bed 30 minutes earlier for extra sleep. Schedule a follow-up with your bariatric medical team. Just keep trying.

This Book's Recipes

The recipes in this book are easy, healthy, and delicious. They require only quick prep and have relatively short cooking times (with the exception, of course, of the slow cooker recipes). You will notice they all follow a familiar pattern. Most are loaded with protein to help you follow the most basic principle of the post-op diet. Most recipes use all whole foods and do not include processed ingredients or obscure pantry items. Many include a variety of fruits and vegetables. Notice the yield for each recipe—many produce big portions intentionally, so you can serve your family and have leftovers for meals later in the week. Nutrition facts are listed for each recipe including grams of fat, protein, carbohydrates, and sugars. Be aware that although the nutrition facts are listed per serving size, your individual portion size may vary, so you may need to adjust accordingly. I've also included recommended servings according to which post-op dietary stage you're in.

Look for these icons in the recipes:

FL full liquid stage   **S** soft foods stage

P puree stage   **G** general diet stage

Focus, too, on the recipe tips, which give ideas about how to enjoy each recipe throughout the stages of your post-op diet. A few basic reminders:

▶ Eat slowly—aim to take 30 minutes to eat a meal.

▶ Avoid drinking with meals. Stop liquid intake for 30 minutes before your meal, and wait 30 minutes after a meal before drinking.

▶ Take your essential vitamin and mineral supplements.

▶ Avoid grazing or mindless snacking.

▶ Be active every day.

▶ Always eat protein-rich foods *first*.

You have all the guidelines you need to achieve weight-loss success. Stay strong and stay true to yourself and your vision for your life after VSG. Stick to the basics, taking it one day at a time, and you are guaranteed to maintain a long-term healthy lifestyle.

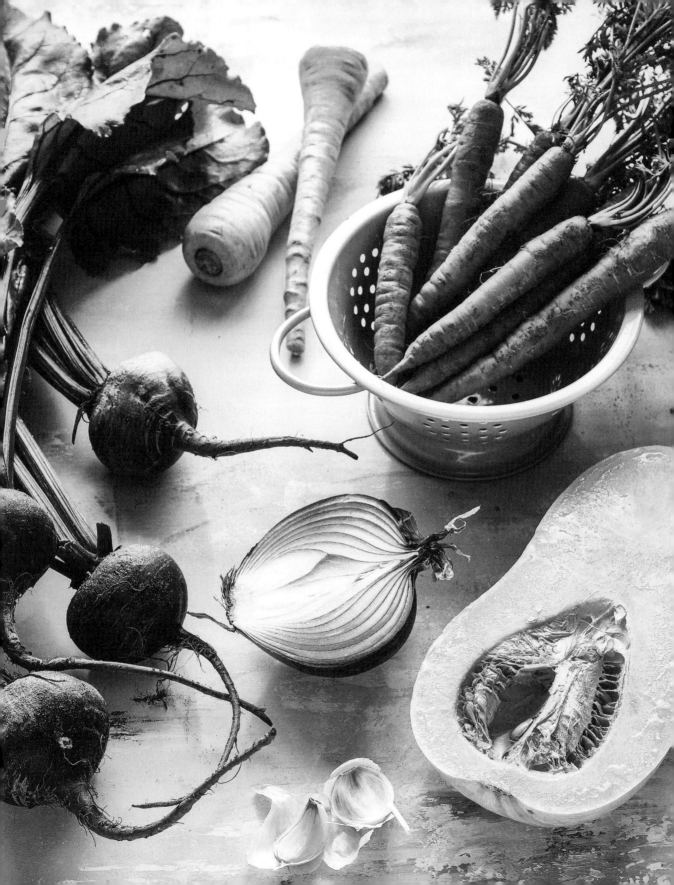

CHAPTER TWO

VSG Meal Plans

Planning meals ahead is a great way to successfully jump-start your post-op diet. After surgery, you may feel overwhelmed with the rapid changes your body is going through and planning meals will be "just one more thing" you have to worry about. But when you know what you are going to eat ahead of time, it makes grocery shopping a breeze and takes away the stress of having nothing to eat when you come home late after work.

Before surgery, many people find they don't plan meals, because they don't have time or it might not be a priority. After surgery, many people forgo planning meals because they aren't interested in food and may not feel hunger. It's important to have a daily plan to get adequate fluids, vitamin supplements, and protein so that you don't miss a meal and end up playing catch-up later. Aim for spreading meals about four to six hours apart, and fit in a glass of High-Protein Milk (page 44) or a protein shake as a snack in between.

A simple tip for meal planning is to cook once and eat the meal at least twice. The majority of recipes in this book contain several servings—enough to feed your entire family and still have leftovers for lunch the next day—and that's intentional. Some recipes can be easily frozen in small servings to eat at a later date. Note that at least one dinner meal per week includes leftovers from a previous meal. Make sure to pull what you need from the freezer a day ahead of time, if necessary. If you find that your household needs fewer servings than the amount the recipes prepare, feel free to save the leftovers and swap them in as another dinner meal during the week to save on food waste and meal prep time.

I hope you will use the following eight weeks of meal plans as a guide to make menu planning easier after surgery. Feel free to swap in your own meal selections depending on your personal preferences and what your schedule allows. Always follow the post-op guidelines as recommended by your surgery center. I strongly urge you to keep track of your grams of daily protein intake. These meal plans are meant to serve as a guide, and since the actual portions you consume may vary, you still need to be mindful of making sure you meet your protein intake. Happy cooking!

WEEK 1 AND WEEK 2
LIQUID DIET Ⓕ🄻

Weeks one and two are all about liquids, liquids, liquids. Staying hydrated is the number one priority in the first two weeks after surgery. Dehydration is one of the most common early complications post-operatively and can have you feeling down and out very quickly. Getting in enough liquids in the early weeks sets the foundation for drinking plenty of water for the long-term, which will help to maximize your weight loss. Here are some other important factors to keep in mind.

▶ When it comes to hydration, focus on getting water in *first* and protein-rich liquids second. Aim for a minimum of 64 ounces of fluid per day from water, other clear liquids, and protein-rich shakes.

▶ Make sure all shakes and smoothies are without seeds or pulp from fruit.

▶ If you are drinking your entire protein shake at mealtimes, you may consider adding High-Protein Milk (page 44) between meals to help increase your protein intake for the day.

▶ Note that each recipe for the protein shakes makes two servings, so refrigerate the second serving for the next day.

WEEK 1 🄵🄻

	BREAKFAST	A.M. SNACK	LUNCH	P.M. SNACK	DINNER
DAY 1	Commercial protein shake with at least 20g protein		Protein-Packed Peanut Butter Cup Shake (page 48)		Double Fudge Chocolate Shake (page 46)
DAY 2	Protein-Packed Peanut Butter Cup Shake (page 48)		Commercial protein shake with at least 20g protein		Double Fudge Chocolate Shake (page 46)
DAY 3	Double Fudge Chocolate Shake (page 46)	Water/calorie-free beverages	Very Vanilla Bean Probiotic Shake (page 47)	Water/calorie-free beverages	Commercial protein shake with at least 20g protein
DAY 4	Commercial protein shake with at least 20g protein		Double Fudge Chocolate Shake (page 46)		Very Vanilla Bean Probiotic Shake (page 47)
DAY 5	Very Vanilla Bean Probiotic Shake (page 47)		Commercial protein shake with at least 20g protein		Protein-Packed Peanut Butter Cup Shake (page 48)
DAY 6	Protein-Packed Peanut Butter Cup Shake (page 48)		Double Fudge Chocolate Shake (page 46)		Commercial protein shake with at least 20g protein
DAY 7	Commercial protein shake with at least 20g protein		Very Vanilla Bean Probiotic Shake (page 47)		Double Fudge Chocolate Shake (page 46)

WEEK 2 FL

	BREAKFAST	A.M. SNACK	LUNCH	P.M. SNACK	DINNER
DAY 1	Double Fudge Chocolate Shake (page 46)	Water/calorie-free beverages/High-Protein Milk (page 44) (optional)	Chunky Monkey Smoothie (page 53)	Water/calorie-free beverages/High-Protein Milk (page 44) (optional)	Commercial protein shake with at least 20g protein
DAY 2	Strawberry-Banana Protein Smoothie (page 54)		Chunky Monkey Smoothie (page 53)		Vanilla Apple Pie Protein Shake (page 49)
DAY 3	Vanilla Apple Pie Protein Shake (page 49)		Commercial protein shake with at least 20g protein		Strawberry-Banana Protein Smoothie (page 54)
DAY 4	Commercial protein shake with at least 20g protein		Berry Blast Protein Shake (page 51)		Double Fudge Chocolate Shake (page 46)
DAY 5	Double Fudge Chocolate Shake (page 46)		Berry Blast Protein Shake (page 51)		Commercial protein shake with at least 20g protein
DAY 6	Pumpkin Spice Latte Protein Shake (page 45)		Tropical Mango Smoothie (page 50)		Very Vanilla Bean Probiotic Shake (page 47)
DAY 7	Pumpkin Spice Latte Protein Shake (page 45)		Very Vanilla Bean Probiotic Shake (page 47)		Tropical Mango Smoothie (page 50)

WEEK 3
PUREED DIET (P)

Pureed foods are slightly thicker in consistency than the liquids you have been consuming to this point and allow you more variety in your diet. Almost anything can be pureed if you have a decent blender or food processor.

▶ During the pureed diet, continue to focus on drinking fluids *first*, getting adequate protein *second*, and supplementing with fruits and vegetables *last*.

▶ Aim for about ¼ to ½ cup of food at each meal. The total volume of food you eat will decrease now that you're switching to more solid foods, since your sleeve will become full more quickly.

▶ Drink High-Protein Milk (page 44) or a protein shake between meals to meet your protein goal.

▶ Use herbs and seasonings to flavor your food—try curry powder, taco seasoning, chili powder, or other seasoning blends (ideally low-sodium) to make pureed foods more interesting.

▶ Use milk, Greek yogurt, water, or broth to thin foods for pureeing to your desired consistency.

▶ Take caution with pureeing foods in catsup, BBQ sauce, or premade sauces, as they can add calories and sugars—check labels carefully.

WEEK 3 ⓟ

	BREAKFAST	A.M. SNACK	LUNCH	P.M. SNACK	DINNER
DAY 1	Best Scrambled Eggs (page 55)	High-Protein Milk (page 44) or protein shake	Classic Tuna Salad (page 56)	High-Protein Milk (page 44) or protein shake	Noodle-less Lasagna with Ricotta Cheese (page 59)
DAY 2	Hearty Slow Cooker Cinnamon Oatmeal (page 63)		Refried Black Beans (page 58) Cottage cheese mixed with taco seasoning		Slow Cooker Barbecue Shredded Chicken (page 135) Mashed Cauliflower (page 76)
DAY 3	Greek yogurt		Classic Tuna Salad (page 56)		Curried Chicken Salad (page 57)
DAY 4	Best Scrambled Eggs (page 55)		Shrimp Cocktail Salad (page 115)		Slow Cooker Barbecue Shredded Chicken (page 135) Mashed Cauliflower (page 76)
DAY 5	Hearty Slow Cooker Cinnamon Oatmeal (page 63)		Classic Tuna Salad (page 56)		Noodle-less Lasagna with Ricotta Cheese (page 59)
DAY 6	Greek yogurt		Curried Chicken Salad (page 57)		Shrimp Cocktail Salad (page 115)
DAY 7	Best Scrambled Eggs (page 55)		Refried Black Beans (page 58) Cottage cheese mixed with taco seasoning		Slow Cooker Barbecue Shredded Chicken (page 135) Mashed Cauliflower (page 76)

WEEK 4
SOAT DIET Ⓢ

As you move from liquids to more solid foods, remember that you may feel fuller quickly and may not be able to eat the full portion of food you planned on eating to meet protein needs. Use High-Protein Milk (page 44), milk, and/or protein shakes between meals to help reach protein goals. Focus on eating food at mealtimes to establish good eating patterns. You may use a protein shake as an occasional meal substitute. Many people find it difficult to eat solid foods in the morning and choose to substitute breakfast with a protein shake on a daily basis.

Portions during this stage will vary. You should be able to eat about 1/2 cup (4 ounces) of food per sitting. Adjust the nutrition fact information according to the portion of food you eat to make sure you are getting adequate protein.

Here are some specific tips for this week's meal plan:

▶ Use leftover chicken from Whole Herbed Roasted Chicken in the Slow Cooker (page 136) to make the Creamy Chicken Soup with Cauliflower (page 121).

▶ Pair steamed/well-cooked vegetables with the Herb-Crusted Salmon (page 108) or Lemon-Parsley Crab Cakes (page 114)—but focus on eating the protein first.

▶ Use canned tuna and crab for the Lemon-Parsley Crab Cakes (page 114), Tuna Noodle-less Casserole (page 106), and Classic Tuna Salad (page 56) to save on prep time, and stock up when it's on sale.

WEEK 4 Ⓢ

	BREAKFAST	A.M. SNACK	LUNCH	P.M. SNACK	DINNER
DAY 1	Wisconsin Scrambler with Aged Cheddar Cheese (page 69)		Classic Tuna Salad (page 56)		Herb-Crusted Salmon (page 108)
DAY 2	Greek yogurt		Herb-Crusted Salmon (page 108)		Whole Herbed Roasted Chicken in the Slow Cooker (page 136)
DAY 3	Wisconsin Scrambler with Aged Cheddar Cheese (page 69)	High-Protein Milk (page 44)/protein shake	Whole Herbed Roasted Chicken in the Slow Cooker (page 136)	High-Protein Milk (page 44)/protein shake	Creamy Chicken Soup with Cauliflower (page 121)
DAY 4	Hearty Slow Cooker Cinnamon Oatmeal (page 63)		Creamy Chicken Soup with Cauliflower (page 121)		Leftovers
DAY 5	Greek yogurt		Cottage cheese with peaches (without skin)		Tuna Noodle-less Casserole (page 106)
DAY 6	Wisconsin Scrambler with Aged Cheddar Cheese (page 69)		Tuna Noodle-less Casserole (page 106)		Slow Cooker Turkey Chili (page 123)
DAY 7	Hearty Slow Cooker Cinnamon Oatmeal (page 63)		Slow Cooker Turkey Chili (page 123)		Lemon-Parsley Crab Cakes (page 114)

WEEK 5
SOFT DIET Ⓢ

You will continue with the soft diet this week. If you are having difficulty meeting your protein needs, you may need to return to a pureed or full liquid diet for a meal or two since you are able to eat a larger volume of food when the food is in liquid form versus soft. For the soft diet, the food consistency should be about what you'd expect when you can easily mash it with a fork. Continue to focus on eating protein foods first, fruits and vegetables second, and all other foods last.

Here are some specific tips for this week's meal plan:

▶ Use leftover chicken from Baked "Fried Chicken" Thighs (page 130) to make the Chicken, Barley, and Vegetable Soup (page 122).

▶ Cut vegetables ahead of time. Allow for meal prep time on the weekend to get food ready for the coming week. Pre-chopped vegetables make dinner prep time during the week a breeze.

▶ While making Roasted Root Vegetables (page 84), bake vegetables for the Roasted Vegetable Quinoa Salad with Chickpeas (page 88).

▶ Save time by preparing the zoodles for Zoodles with Turkey Meatballs (page 134) and zucchini for Mexican Taco Skillet with Red Peppers and Zucchini (page 140). Try rolling the meatballs for the spaghetti dish while browning the ground turkey for the taco skillet.

WEEK 5 ⑤

	BREAKFAST	A.M. SNACK	LUNCH	P.M. SNACK	DINNER
DAY 1	High-Protein Pancakes (page 65)	High-Protein Milk (page 44)/protein shake	Lemon-Parsley Crab Cakes (page 114)	High-Protein Milk (page 44)/protein shake	Eggplant Rollatini (page 96)
DAY 2	Farmer's Egg Casserole with Broccoli, Mushroom, and Onions (page 72)		Eggplant Rollatini (page 96)		Baked "Fried Chicken" Thighs (page 130) Roasted Root Vegetables (page 84)
DAY 3	High-Protein Pancakes (page 65)		Baked "Fried Chicken" Thighs (page 130) Roasted Root Vegetables (page 84)		Roasted Vegetable Quinoa Salad with Chickpeas (page 88)
DAY 4	Farmer's Egg Casserole with Broccoli, Mushroom, and Onions (page 72)		Roasted Vegetable Quinoa Salad with Chickpeas (page 88)		Chicken, Barley, and Vegetable Soup (page 122)
DAY 5	High-Protein Pancakes (page 65)		Chicken, Barley, and Vegetable Soup (page 122)		Mexican Taco Skillet with Red Peppers and Zucchini (page 140)
DAY 6	Greek yogurt		Mexican Taco Skillet with Red Peppers and Zucchini (page 140)		Leftovers
DAY 7	Farmer's Egg Casserole with Broccoli, Mushroom, and Onions (page 72)		Cottage cheese with fruit		Zoodles with Turkey Meatballs (page 134)

WEEK 6
SOFT DIET ⓢ

Before you begin this week, reflect on how much protein you've been eating. Check your protein goal. Are you hitting it with your meals and two cups of milk per day? Slowly wind down the use of protein shakes and/or High-Protein Milk (page 44) as you are able to eat more solid proteins from food. Use the "snacks" between meals to supplement total protein intake as needed, but be careful not to add unnecessary calories.

Portions during this stage will vary. You should be able to eat about ½ cup (4 ounces) of food per sitting. Make sure to adjust the nutrition fact information according to the portion of food you eat to make sure you are getting adequate protein.

Here are some specific tips for this week's meal plan:

▶ Toss together the ingredients for Slow Cooker White Chicken Chili (page 124) ahead of time in a large gallon-size freezer bag, and pull it out later in the week to toss in the slow cooker.

▶ Consider mixing up your Mediterranean Turkey Meatloaf (page 138) ahead of time and freezing it or baking it in advance to save on preparation time the day you want to eat it.

▶ Keep your fish fresh. Prepare fish dinners on the day of and eat leftovers within one or two days. Consider reheating fish in the oven (not the microwave), or eating it cold, to keep it from developing the rubbery texture that can happen if it's overheated.

WEEK 6 Ⓢ

	BREAKFAST	A.M. SNACK	LUNCH	P.M. SNACK	DINNER
DAY 1	Best Scrambled Eggs (page 55)		Zoodles with Turkey Meatballs (page 134)		Seafood Cioppino (page 116)
DAY 2	Cherry-Vanilla Baked Oatmeal (page 64)		Seafood Cioppino (page 116)		Italian Eggplant Pizzas (page 80)
DAY 3	Greek yogurt	1 cup milk/High-Protein Milk (page 44)/protein shake	Italian Eggplant Pizzas (page 80)	1 cup milk/High-Protein Milk (page 44)/protein shake	Red Snapper Veracruz (page 113)
DAY 4	Cherry-Vanilla Baked Oatmeal (page 64)		Red Snapper Veracruz (page 113)		Leftovers
DAY 5	Best Scrambled Eggs (page 55)		Cottage cheese with fruit		Slow Cooker White Chicken Chili (page 124)
DAY 6	Greek yogurt		Slow Cooker White Chicken Chili (page 124)		Fried-less Friday Fish Fry with Cod (page 111) Baked Zucchini Fries (page 79)
DAY 7	Cherry-Vanilla Baked Oatmeal (page 64)		Fried-less Friday Fish Fry with Cod (page 111) Baked Zucchini Fries (page 79)		Mediterranean Turkey Meatloaf (page 138)

GENERAL DIET Ⓖ

This week is exciting, as the food you can now eat continues to be more diverse in texture. Although you may be ready to put the blender and food processor aside in place of eating "regular" food again, be sensitive to your sleeve. You may need to swap in a protein shake for a meal here or there, depending on what your body is tolerating. Stress, lack of sleep, and illness are all factors that may influence what you can tolerate on any given day.

Here are some specific tips for this week's meal plan:

▶ Make the Mexican Stuffed Summer Squash (page 90) ahead of time. Bake it on the day you plan to eat it to shorten meal prep time.

▶ Prep your chicken once for two meals. While baking the Chicken Cordon Bleu (page 133), prepare the chicken for the next day's Chicken "Nachos" with Sweet Bell Peppers (page 127).

WEEK 7 ⓖ

	BREAKFAST	A.M. SNACK	LUNCH	P.M. SNACK	DINNER
DAY 1	Southwestern Scrambled Egg Burritos (page 71)		Mediterranean Turkey Meatloaf (page 138)		Baked Halibut with Tomatoes and White Wine (page 110)
DAY 2	Greek yogurt		Baked Halibut with Tomatoes and White Wine (page 110)		Coconut Curry Tofu Bowl (page 94)
DAY 3	Southwestern Scrambled Egg Burritos (page 71)	1 cup milk/High-Protein Milk (page 44)	Coconut Curry Tofu Bowl (page 94)	1 cup milk/High-Protein Milk (page 44)	Mexican Stuffed Summer Squash (page 90)
DAY 4	Andrea's Hangry Eggs with Cauliflower (page 70)		Mexican Stuffed Summer Squash (page 90)		Leftovers
DAY 5	Smoothie Bowl with Greek Yogurt and Fresh Berries (page 62)		Cottage Cheese with fruit		Chicken Cordon Bleu (page 133)
DAY 6	Andrea's Hangry Eggs with Cauliflower (page 70)		Chicken Cordon Bleu (page 133)		Chicken "Nachos" with Sweet Bell Peppers (page 127)
DAY 7	Smoothie Bowl with Greek Yogurt and Fresh Berries (page 62)		Chicken "Nachos" with Sweet Bell Peppers (page 127)		Classic Tuna Salad (page 56)

GENERAL DIET Ⓖ

Congratulations! You have made it to week 8. The first two months following your sleeve gastrectomy are the most restrictive diet-wise. By week 8, you should be ready to progress to a diet with more variety and that's more reflective of the types of foods you could eat before surgery. Portions during this stage will vary. You should be able to eat up to 1 cup of food per sitting. Adjust the nutrition fact information according to the portion of food you eat to ensure you are getting adequate protein. If you feel that you aren't tolerating the foods in the continued general diet, go back and repeat an earlier week's diet, and then try to add these foods again in another week or two.

Continue to drink 1 cup of milk between meals for snacks. Depending on the day, you may need to swap in a protein shake and/or High-Protein Milk (page 44) to make sure you meet your protein needs. As time goes on, try to drink plain 1% or nonfat milk to make it easy, save on cost, and forgo added unnecessary calories from protein supplements, since you can now meet your protein goals with whole foods.

Here are some specific tips for this week's meal plan:

▶ Add some steamed vegetables on the side of your Slow-Roasted Pesto Salmon (page 109).

▶ Make sure you have plenty extra Ranch-Seasoned Crispy Chicken Tenders (page 126) to use for your Buffalo Chicken Wrap (page 128).

▶ Prep your Butternut Squash and Black Bean Enchiladas (page 102) on the weekend to save time on meal prep later in the week.

▶ Prep your Cheesy Cauliflower Casserole (page 100) ahead of time and freeze any leftovers—this could be a quick lunch on its own.

WEEK 8 ⓖ

	BREAKFAST	A.M. SNACK	LUNCH	P.M. SNACK	DINNER
DAY 1	Hard-boiled Eggs and Avocado on Toast (page 68)	1 cup milk/High-Protein Milk (page 44)	Classic Tuna Salad (page 56)	1 cup milk/High-Protein Milk (page 44)	Slow-Roasted Pesto Salmon (page 109)
DAY 2	Hearty Slow Cooker Cinnamon Oatmeal (page 63)		Slow-Roasted Pesto Salmon (page 109)		Leftovers
DAY 3	Hard-boiled Eggs and Avocado on Toast (page 68)		Cottage cheese and fruit		Ranch-Seasoned Crispy Chicken Tenders (page 126) Cheesy Cauliflower Casserole (page 100)
DAY 4	Hearty Slow Cooker Cinnamon Oatmeal (page 63)		Ranch-Seasoned Crispy Chicken Tenders (page 126) Cheesy Cauliflower Casserole (page 100)		Butternut Squash and Black Bean Enchiladas (page 102)
DAY 5	High-Protein Pancakes (page 65)		Butternut Squash and Black Bean Enchiladas (page 102)		Buffalo Chicken Wrap (page 128)
DAY 6	Greek yogurt		Buffalo Chicken Wrap (page 128)		Cauliflower Pizza with Caramelized Onions and Chicken Sausage (page 142)
DAY 7	High-Protein Pancakes (page 65)		Cauliflower Pizza with Caramelized Onions and Chicken Sausage (page 142)		Dinner out at restaurant—order fish and cooked vegetables

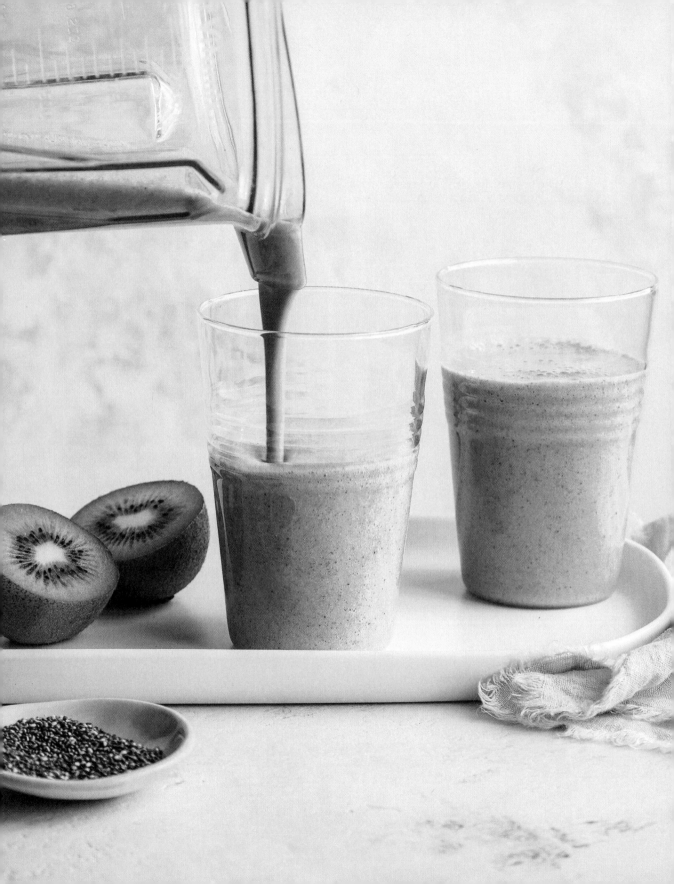

CHAPTER THREE

Early Post-Op Foods

High-Protein Milk

MAKES 4 SERVINGS / PREP TIME: 5 MINUTES / TOTAL TIME: 5 MINUTES

If you have read my first cookbook, Fresh Start Bariatric Cookbook, you are familiar with my go-to recipe for High-Protein Milk. It will cost you only about 40 cents per cup to make, and it brings in a whopping 14 grams of protein! It's a reminder that getting in your protein doesn't have to be complicated with fancy protein powders. Use this recipe to make a batch to drink by itself, use as a base for protein shakes, or in milk for cooking. This drink should be a part of everyone's recipe box after a sleeve gastrectomy.

4 cups skim milk
1 cup nonfat dry
  milk powder

Post-Op Servings

 1 cup, as many times per day as needed to reach protein goal

1 to 3 cups per day

1 In a deep bowl or a blender, beat the milk and milk powder slowly with a beater or blend on high speed to mix for about 5 minutes, until the powder is well dissolved and no longer visible.

2 Refrigerate any milk you don't drink or use right away in an airtight container. The flavor improves overnight. Discard any remaining milk after 7 days.

Did You Know? *Milk is a great source of protein, vitamins, and minerals essential for healing and weight loss after surgery. Plant-based milks such as almond, rice, hemp, and coconut milk may be nutrient dense but lack the rich protein content of cow's milk. Soy milk has a protein content similar to cow's milk at 6 to 7 grams per cup. All milk products contain some natural sugar. Milk contains lactose, which is different from foods and beverages that contain added sugars. Lactose is a disaccharide your body needs to break down in order to digest and absorb it. People who have lactose intolerance should choose lactose-free milk or take lactase enzymes when they eat dairy products to help digest this sugar.*

Per Serving (1 cup): Calories: 144; Total fat: 0g; Protein 14g; Carbs: 21g; Fiber: 0g; Sugar: 21g; Sodium: 218mg

Pumpkin Spice Latte Protein Shake

MAKES 2 SERVINGS / PREP TIME: 5 MINUTES / TOTAL TIME: 5 MINUTES

Imagine the fall season all wrapped up into one beverage. Heartwarming coffee, sweet pumpkin, aromatic cinnamon, and nutmeg—this protein shake is sure to meet your autumn craving for a pumpkin-spiced latte from your favorite coffee shop, but without all the added sugar and fat.

1 cup low-fat milk or
   unsweetened soy milk
½ cup pumpkin puree
1 scoop (¼ cup) vanilla
   protein powder
¾ cup brewed
   decaf coffee
1 teaspoon ground
   cinnamon
¼ teaspoon ground ginger
¼ teaspoon
   ground nutmeg
⅛ teaspoon ground cloves

Post-Op Servings

1 to 3 cups per day

1   In a blender, combine the milk, pumpkin puree, protein powder, coffee, cinnamon, ginger, nutmeg, and cloves and blend on high for 2 to 3 minutes, until the shake is smooth and the powder is well dissolved.

2   Pour half the shake into a glass and enjoy.

3   Refrigerate any shake you don't drink or use right away in an airtight container for up to 1 week. Reblend prior to serving.

Cooking tip: *Make your own pumpkin pie spice. Add it to smoothies, oatmeal, and baked squash, or to flavor plain Greek yogurt. Combine 2 tablespoons ground cinnamon, 1 teaspoon ground ginger, 1 teaspoon ground nutmeg, 1/2 teaspoon ground cloves, and 1/2 teaspoon ground allspice. Store in an airtight container.*

Per Serving (1 cup): Calories: 125; Total fat: 0g; Protein: 15g; Carbs: 12g; Fiber: 2g; Sugar: 8g; Sodium: 155mg

Double Fudge Chocolate Shake

MAKES 2 SERVINGS / PREP TIME: 5 MINUTES / TOTAL TIME: 5 MINUTES

Chocolate. Some people love it so much they put it in its own food group—fruits, vegetables, protein, grains, dairy, and chocolate. Having a sleeve gastrectomy means giving up a lot of rich desserts, but it doesn't mean you have to entirely give up this delicious treat. Try unsweetened cocoa powder in smoothies, shakes, and yogurt for chocolate flavor without added sugars.

1 cup low-fat milk or unsweetened soy milk

½ cup low-fat plain Greek yogurt

1 scoop (¼ cup) chocolate protein powder

2 tablespoons unsweetened cocoa powder

½ small banana

½ teaspoon vanilla extract

1 In a blender, combine the milk, yogurt, protein powder, cocoa powder, banana, and vanilla and blend on high speed for 2 to 3 minutes, until the shake is smooth and the powders are well dissolved.

2 Pour half the shake into a glass and enjoy.

3 Refrigerate any shake you don't drink or use right away in an airtight container for up to 1 week. Reblend prior to serving.

Post-Op Servings

1 to 3 cups per day

Ingredient tip: *Chocolate is made from the cocoa (or cacao) bean. You can find two versions of baking cocoa in your grocery store—Dutch-process cocoa powder or unsweetened cocoa powder. Look for 100 percent unsweetened cocoa powder, which is slightly more acidic in taste than the Dutch-process version, but richer in heart-healthy antioxidants and flavonols. When baking, pay attention to which version is called for in a recipe as the type of cocoa powder you choose can have a leavening effect on your baked goods.*

Per Serving (1 cup): Calories: 157; Total fat: 1g; Protein: 20g; Carbs: 18g; Fiber: 3g; Sugar: 8g; Sodium: 156mg

Very Vanilla Bean Probiotic Shake

MAKES 2 SERVINGS / PREP TIME: 5 MINUTES / TOTAL TIME: 5 MINUTES

Not all bacteria are created alike. Our gastrointestinal tract is loaded with both good and not-so-good bacteria. Whether our bodies are in good microbial balance can affect our health. In fact, research shows that the type of bacteria found in the intestinal tract of normal weight versus obese individuals can be different. Including foods rich in probiotics or healthy bacteria may help promote overall good health—especially pertaining to gut health. Try this creamy vanilla protein shake made with kefir—a fermented milk drink that is lactose-free and packed with more healthy bacteria than your typical cup of yogurt.

1 cup unsweetened vanilla soy milk or low-fat milk

1 scoop (¼ cup) vanilla protein powder

½ cup low-fat plain kefir

¼ cup low-fat plain Greek yogurt

1 teaspoon vanilla extract

5 ice cubes

Post-Op Servings

1 to 3 cups per day

1 In a blender, combine the milk, protein powder, kefir, yogurt, vanilla, and ice cubes. Blend on high speed for 3 to 4 minutes, or until the powder is well dissolved and no longer visible.

2 Pour half the shake into a glass and enjoy.

3 Refrigerate any shake you don't drink or use right away in an airtight container for up to 1 week. Reblend prior to serving.

Ingredient tip: *Look for kefir in the dairy section of your grocery store near the yogurt. Mix low-fat plain kefir into overnight oatmeal, shakes, and smoothies. Have caution with flavored versions of kefir as they are loaded with lots of added sugars. Look for varieties sweetened with stevia to save on calories.*

Per Serving (1 cup): Calories: 153; Total fat: 3g; Protein: 22g; Carbs: 8g; Fiber: 2g; Sugar: 6g; Sodium: 161mg

Protein-Packed Peanut Butter Cup Shake

MAKES 2 SERVINGS / PREP TIME: 5 MINUTES / TOTAL TIME: 5 MINUTES

It may be no surprise to you that Reese's Peanut Butter Cups are one of the top-selling candies in the world. The creamy peanut butter filling surrounded by sweet chocolate is a treat that's hard for most to pass up. Although those peanut butter cups are off limits after surgery, this creamy shake is sure to meet your craving and provide plenty of protein. Try this as an afternoon snack to fix your sweet tooth and ward off grazing at the office candy jar.

1 cup low-fat milk

½ cup low-fat plain Greek yogurt

¼ cup nonfat ricotta cheese

1 scoop (¼ cup) chocolate protein powder

2 tablespoons powdered peanut butter

2 tablespoons cocoa powder

Post-Op Servings

1 to 3 cups per day

1 In a blender, combine the milk, yogurt, ricotta, protein powder, powdered peanut butter, and cocoa powder. Blend on high speed for 3 to 4 minutes, until the powders are well dissolved and no longer visible.

2 Pour half the shake into a glass and enjoy.

3 Refrigerate any shake you don't drink or use right away in an airtight container for up to 1 week. Reblend prior to serving.

Post-op tip: *Although peanut butter is packed with heart-healthy fat, it's loaded with calories as well. Be mindful of portions as 1 tablespoon brings in a whopping 90 calories. When eating regular peanut butter after surgery, be sure to choose natural versions without added palm oil (a saturated fat) or added sugars. Mix and store upside down in the fridge to keep it emulsified. As an alternative, you can also mix powdered peanut butter with water to turn it into a creamy spread for toast or adding to oatmeal. Powdered peanut butter is loaded with protein but without excess calories from fat.*

Per Serving (1 cup): Calories: 215; Total fat: 3g; Protein: 27g; Carbs: 18g; Fiber: 3g; Sugar: 11g; Sodium: 249mg

Vanilla Apple Pie Protein Shake

MAKES 2 SERVINGS / PREP TIME: 5 MINUTES / TOTAL TIME: 5 MINUTES

Nothing feels more comforting than fresh apple pie with ice cream. This classic dessert brings feelings of warmth from Mom's or Grandma's house. Whip up this apple pie–flavored shake to taste the comfort of apple pie in a drink that is low enough in calories to keep trimming your waistline.

1 cup low-fat milk

1 scoop (¼ cup) vanilla protein powder

1 small apple, peeled, cored, and chopped

1 teaspoon vanilla extract

2 teaspoons ground cinnamon

½ teaspoon ground nutmeg

5 ice cubes

Post-Op Servings

1 to 3 cups per day

1 In a blender, combine the milk, protein powder, apple, vanilla, cinnamon, nutmeg, and ice cubes. Blend on high speed for 3 to 4 minutes, until the powder is well dissolved and no longer visible.

2 Pour half the shake into a glass and enjoy.

3 Refrigerate any shake you don't drink or use right away in an airtight container for up to 1 week. Reblend prior to serving.

Per Serving (1 cup): Calories: 123; Total fat: 1g; Protein: 14g; Carbs: 14g; Fiber: 1g; Sugar: 12g; Sodium: 153mg

Tropical Mango Smoothie

MAKES 2 SERVINGS / PREP TIME: 5 MINUTES / TOTAL TIME: 5 MINUTES

Whether poolside, beachside, or simply relaxing in your very own backyard—fruit smoothies are refreshing on a hot summer day. Without thinking twice, you may quickly drink several hundred calories from these types of sugary beverages—often not made from 100 percent fruit. Try this recipe for a lighter fruit smoothie that will have you feeling like you have been swept away to a tropical beach destination.

1 cup unsweetened coconut milk or low-fat milk

1 scoop (¼ cup) vanilla protein powder

¼ cup frozen mango chunks

¼ cup canned pineapple chunks in 100% natural juice or water, drained

½ cup low-fat plain Greek yogurt

5 ice cubes

Post-Op Servings

1 to 3 cups per day

1 In a blender, combine the milk, protein powder, mango, pineapple, yogurt, and ice cubes. Blend on high speed for 3 to 4 minutes, until the powder is well dissolved and no longer visible.

2 Pour half the smoothie into a glass and enjoy.

3 Refrigerate any shake you don't drink or use right away in an airtight container for up to 1 week. Reblend prior to serving.

Ingredient tip: *Shop for fruit in the freezer section of the grocery store. Frozen fruit adds to the desired thick consistency of a smoothie or protein shake without having to add additional ice cubes. It can save you money when you're buying fruits that may not be in season. And you don't have to worry about the fruit going bad before you use it since it holds its own in the freezer for months at a time. Just make sure you buy only 100 percent pure fruit without any added sugars.*

Per Serving (1 cup): Calories: 115; Total fat: 2.5g; Protein: 15g; Carbs: 9g; Fiber: 1g; Sugar: 7g; Sodium: 136mg

Berry Blast Protein Shake

MAKES 2 SERVINGS / PREP TIME: 5 MINUTES / TOTAL TIME: 5 MINUTES

It's no secret that berries are loaded with some of the highest content of antioxidants—more than almost any other fruit. Berries are loaded with fiber, low in calories, and rich in vitamin C. Mixed frozen berries pack in phytochemicals and a blast of natural color. No artificial flavorings or red dye here!

1 cup low-fat milk or unsweetened soy milk

¾ cup mixed frozen berries

1 scoop (¼ cup) vanilla or plain protein powder

5 ice cubes

Post-Op Servings

1 to 3 cups per day

1 In a blender, combine the milk, berries, protein powder, and ice cubes. Blend on high speed for 3 to 4 minutes, until the powder is well dissolved and no longer visible.

2 Pour half the shake into a glass and enjoy.

3 Refrigerate any shake you don't drink or use right away in an airtight container for up to 1 week. Reblend prior to serving.

Per Serving (1 cup): Calories: 126; Total fat: 1g; Protein: 15g; Carbs: 14g; Fiber: 3g; Sugar: 10g; Sodium: 153mg

Spinach Superfood Smoothie

MAKES 2 SERVINGS / PREP TIME: 5 MINUTES / TOTAL TIME: 5 MINUTES

Some health food companies sell greens blends with lots of herbal additives and claims that consumption will protect against various health conditions. Not only are these blends expensive, but in order to maximize the protective health benefits of eating fruits and vegetables you must also consume the whole food—not a supplement. Get in your greens from the original source by trying this smoothie loaded with fresh spinach, kiwi, and cucumber. It's sweetened with fresh banana, and it's got some power-packed flax and chia seeds in it, too, for good measure.

1 cup fresh spinach

1 kiwi fruit, peeled and cut into chunks

½ medium cucumber, peeled

½ small banana

1 cup unsweetened almond milk or low-fat milk

1 tablespoon ground flaxseed

1 teaspoon chia seeds

1 scoop (¼ cup) unflavored or vanilla protein powder

10 to 12 ice cubes

1 In a blender, add the spinach, kiwi, cucumber, banana, milk, flaxseed, chia seeds, protein powder, and ice cubes. Blend on high speed for 2 to 3 minutes, until the shake is smooth and no longer lumpy. If the shake is too thick, blend in 2 to 4 tablespoons of water to reach your desired consistency.

2 Pour half the shake into a glass and enjoy.

3 Refrigerate any shake you don't drink or use right away in an airtight container for up to 1 week. Reblend prior to serving.

Per Serving (1 cup): Calories 148; Total fat 4g; Protein: 13g; Carbs: 17g; Fiber: 5g; Sugar: 7g; Sodium: 193 mg

Post-Op Servings

 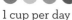

1 cup per day

Chunky Monkey Smoothie

MAKES 2 SERVINGS / PREP TIME: 5 MINUTES / TOTAL TIME: 5 MINUTES

After surgery, you won't be sitting down to a pint of Ben & Jerry's ice cream, but that doesn't mean you have to sacrifice the Chunky Monkey combo of fudgy chocolate and banana. Try this smoothie to get plenty of protein in a creamy smoothie without all the sugar and fat in the ice cream version.

1 small banana, frozen

1 cup unsweetened almond milk

½ cup low-fat plain Greek yogurt

1 scoop (¼ cup) chocolate protein powder

2 tablespoons powdered peanut butter

1 cup ice cubes

1 In a blender, combine the banana, milk, yogurt, protein powder, powdered peanut butter, and ice cubes. Blend on high speed for 2 to 3 minutes, until the shake is smooth and there are no lumps.

2 Pour half the shake into a glass and enjoy.

3 Refrigerate any shake you don't drink or use right away in an airtight container for up to 1 week. Reblend prior to serving.

Post-Op Servings

1 cup per day

Serving tip: *Toss fresh over-ripened bananas in the freezer instead of the garbage. Use them for baking—you can even substitute them for oil in many recipes. Or add them to a smoothie like this one. Note that the banana will further brown upon freezing but may taste even sweeter than when fresh!*

Per Serving (1 cup): Calories 194; Total fat 4g; Protein: 20g; Carbs: 23g; Fiber: 4g; Sugar: 11g; Sodium: 245 mg

Strawberry-Banana Protein Smoothie

MAKES 2 SERVINGS / PREP TIME: 5 MINUTES / TOTAL TIME: 5 MINUTES

Banana split—reboot! This smoothie will remind you of buttery vanilla ice cream topped with delish fresh strawberries and banana. In fact, the bananas add the perfect creamy texture. Keep a bag of frozen strawberries in your freezer so you'll always have the ingredients available.

1 cup low-fat milk

1 scoop (¼ cup) vanilla or unflavored protein powder

⅓ ripe banana

½ cup frozen strawberries

5 ice cubes

Post-Op Servings

1 to 3 cups per day

1 In a blender, blend on high speed to combine the milk, protein powder, banana, frozen strawberries, and ice cubes for 3 to 4 minutes, until the powders are well dissolved and no longer visible.

2 Pour half of the shake into a glass and enjoy.

3 Refrigerate any shake you don't drink or use right away in an airtight container for up to 1 week. Reblend prior to serving.

Ingredient tip: *Only use one-third of a banana to help save on calories and sugars, since bananas can be particularly dense in carbohydrates. Save leftover banana for the next day or toss in the freezer and use for baking muffins at a later date.*

Per Serving (1 cup): Calories: 131; Total fat: 1g; Protein: 16g; Carbs: 14g; Fiber: 2g; Sugar: 11g; Sodium: 154 mg

Best Scrambled Eggs

MAKES 2 SERVINGS / PREP TIME: 5 MINUTES / COOK TIME: 15 MINUTES
TOTAL TIME: 20 MINUTES

Eggs are a diet staple after the sleeve gastrectomy. They contain high-quality protein, they're low in calories, they're easy to make for a quick meal, and they're gentler on your sleeve than more dense meat sources of protein. Most of us know the basics for making scrambled eggs, but check out the post-op tips for ideas to add more flavor to typical scrambled eggs and suggestions for how to add more protein.

Nonstick cooking spray
2 large eggs
1 tablespoon low-fat milk
½ teaspoon dried thyme
Freshly ground
    black pepper

Post-Op Servings

P ¼ cup or 1 egg

S ½ cup or 2 eggs

G 2 eggs

1 Coat the bottom of a small skillet with the cooking spray and place over medium heat.

2 In a small bowl, beat the eggs lightly with a fork or whisk. Beat in the milk and thyme.

3 Add the egg mixture to the skillet, and reduce the heat to medium-low. Stir the eggs gently and constantly with a rubber spatula for 10 to 15 minutes, until fluffy and cooked thoroughly.

4 Grind some black pepper over the eggs and enjoy.

Post-op tip: *After cooking, toss these eggs in the blender to eat on the pureed diet. Eat them immediately while they are still warm. Consider adding 1 tablespoon powdered egg whites to the egg-and-milk mixture for additional protein. Mix well to dissolve the egg white powder, and you will never know it's there as the taste does not change. You can add cheese for additional protein as well. When you advance to a soft diet or general-consistency diet, add chunks of nitrate-free deli meat or shredded chicken to continue to add more protein. Additional seasonings to improve the flavor in your eggs include rosemary, chives, or dill, or top them with salsa or hot sauce.*

Per Serving (¼ cup): Calories: 87; Total fat: 6g; Protein: 7g; Carbs: 1g; Fiber: 0g; Sugar: 0g; Sodium: 83mg

Classic Tuna Salad

MAKES 3 SERVINGS / PREP TIME: 10 MINUTES / TOTAL TIME: 10 MINUTES

It's no wonder fish and seafood are perfect staples for any weight-loss plan—they are loaded with protein and extremely low in calories. Because they are generally soft and much less dense than meat protein, they are a great addition to your post-op meal plan. Canned tuna is inexpensive, not to mention extremely convenient and well tolerated after surgery. Add a bit of fresh lemon, onion, and pickle relish for a delish flavor combination.

1 (5-ounce) can water-packed tuna

1 tablespoon freshly squeezed lemon juice

1 tablespoon olive oil-based mayonnaise

1 tablespoon low-fat plain Greek yogurt

½ teaspoon Dijon mustard

1 tablespoon finely chopped red onion

1 teaspoon pickle relish or finely chopped pickles

½ teaspoon freshly ground black pepper

Post-Op Servings

P ¼ cup

S ½ cup

G ½ to 1 cup

1 In a fine mesh sieve, drain the tuna over the sink. Transfer it to a small bowl.

2 Add the lemon juice, mayonnaise, Greek yogurt, Dijon mustard, red onion, pickle relish, and black pepper and mix with the tuna until well combined.

3 Serve right away or cover and refrigerate overnight to improve the flavors.

Ingredient tip: *Tuna salad doesn't have to be boring or one-note. Variations abound to keep it exciting and flavorful. To add healthy fat, swap the mayo for avocado. To deepen flavor, mix plain tuna with powdered ranch salad dressing. To boost protein, mix with cottage cheese (plus a little salt and pepper) for a puree-friendly meal. To add texture on a general diet, stir in chopped fresh apple and sunflower seeds. To vary presentation, serve in a hollowed-out tomato, bell pepper, or cantaloupe.*

Per Serving (¼ cup): Calories: 73; Total fat: 2g; Protein: 11g; Carbs: 3g; Fiber: 0g; Sugar: 1g; Sodium: 261 mg

Curried Chicken Salad

MAKES 7 SERVINGS / PREP TIME: 10 MINUTES / TOTAL TIME: 10 MINUTES

Although many people steer away from eating meat after surgery because it's extremely filling and dense, serving it with a moist sauce can help make it easier to digest. Chicken salad is one of those examples. Traditional chicken salads are laden with loads of high-calorie mayonnaise. This recipe is packed with curry-inspired flavors to jazz up boring old chicken salad, and healthier Greek yogurt is mixed with a natural mayonnaise to create a creamy and tasty finished product. Make sure to check the ingredients list on the mayonnaise—for a natural version, you'll want to see olive oil, not soybean oil.

2 tablespoons low-fat plain Greek yogurt

1 tablespoon olive oil-based mayonnaise

1 tablespoon freshly squeezed lemon juice

1 teaspoon curry powder

1½ cups diced cooked chicken or 1 (12.5-ounce) can chicken breast

Post-Op Servings

P ¼ cup

S ½ cup

G ½ to 1 cup

1 In a medium bowl, mix together the yogurt, mayonnaise, lemon juice, and curry powder until well combined.

2 Add the chicken to the bowl and mix until everything is well combined and all the chicken is coated.

3 Serve right away or cover and refrigerate overnight to improve the flavors.

Ingredient tip: *On a general diet, serve this dish with different add-ins. To boost fiber and sweetness, add golden raisins or quartered grapes. To enhance flavor, add fresh herbs such as scallions. (To save prep time, use scissors instead of a knife to cut those fresh herbs!) To add texture, stir in chopped, slivered almonds.*

Per Serving (¼ cup): Calories: 84; Total fat: 2g; Protein: 16g; Carbs: 1g; Fiber: 0g; Sugar: 0g; Sodium: 43mg

Refried Black Beans

MAKES 4 SERVINGS / PREP TIME: 10 MINUTES / COOK TIME: 5 MINUTES
TOTAL TIME: 15 MINUTES

Vegetarian refried beans are a great source of protein and fiber—two nutrients needed after surgery in high amounts. Pantry staple alert: Beans are a wonderfully inexpensive protein source; keep cans of beans on hand for the early days after surgery or simply to make a meal in a hurry at any time. Most refried bean recipes are made with pinto beans; try this alternative version with black beans for the same great benefits with a unique twist.

1 teaspoon extra-virgin olive oil

1 teaspoon minced garlic

1 (15-ounce) can black beans, drained and rinsed

1 tablespoon freshly squeezed lime juice

1 teaspoon smoked paprika

½ teaspoon dried oregano

¼ teaspoon cayenne pepper

½ teaspoon ground cumin

Post-Op Servings

Ⓟ ¼ cup

Ⓢ ½ cup

Ⓖ ½ to 1 cup

1 In a small pot over medium-low heat, heat the olive oil and add the garlic. Stir for 1 minute. Add the beans and cook until warm throughout, about 5 minutes. Turn off the heat. Add the lime juice, paprika, oregano, cayenne, and cumin, and mix to combine.

2 To reach the desired consistency, use a blender or immersion blender to puree the beans, or mash them with a potato masher.

Post-op tip: *These tasty refried beans are perfect for the pureed stage post-op. Stir in some powdered egg whites or unflavored protein powder to increase your protein load for the meal. You can also add some cheese for extra flavor and protein—try Monterey Jack or an aged Cheddar.*

Per Serving (¼ cup): Calories: 121; Total fat: 1g; Protein: 7g; Carbs: 20g; Fiber: 7g; Sugar: 0g; Sodium: 2mg

Noodle-less Lasagna with Ricotta Cheese

MAKES 8 SERVINGS / PREP TIME: 10 MINUTES / COOK TIME: 20 MINUTES
TOTAL TIME: 30 MINUTES

Italian food means comfort, and nothing says comfort food like lasagna. Noodles may be out of the question right after surgery, but this creamy ricotta cheese topped with sauce will have you thinking you just ate a serving of rich, cheesy lasagna.

Nonstick cooking spray

1 (15-ounce) container part-skim ricotta cheese

¼ cup grated Parmigiano-Reggiano cheese

1 large egg, lightly beaten

½ cup Marinara Sauce with Italian Herbs (page 178) or a low-sugar jarred marinara sauce

½ cup shredded part-skim mozzarella cheese

Post-Op Servings

P ¼ cup

S ½ cup

G ½ to 1 cup

1 Preheat the oven to 375°F. Coat an 8-by-8 baking dish with the cooking spray.

2 In a small bowl, combine the ricotta cheese, Parmigiano-Reggiano cheese, and egg.

3 Spread the cheese mixture over the bottom of the baking dish.

4 Layer the marinara sauce over the ricotta mixture and top it with the mozzarella cheese.

5 Bake for 15 to 20 minutes or until the mozzarella cheese is bubbly.

Ingredient tip: *Ricotta and cottage cheese are excellent sources of protein, and the skim and part-skim versions are low in calories. Plus, they are extremely well tolerated in the first few days and weeks post-op. There are any numbers of ways to add different flavors to each. For a sweet ricotta treat, mix it with some cinnamon, vanilla extract, and stevia. For a more savory dish, stir some dried onions and chives into your cottage cheese. You can even head to the Southwest by stirring some taco seasoning into your cottage cheese!*

Per Serving (¼ cup): Calories: 121; Total fat: 7g; Protein: 9g; Carbs: 6g; Fiber: 0g; Sugar: 2g; Sodium: 234 mg

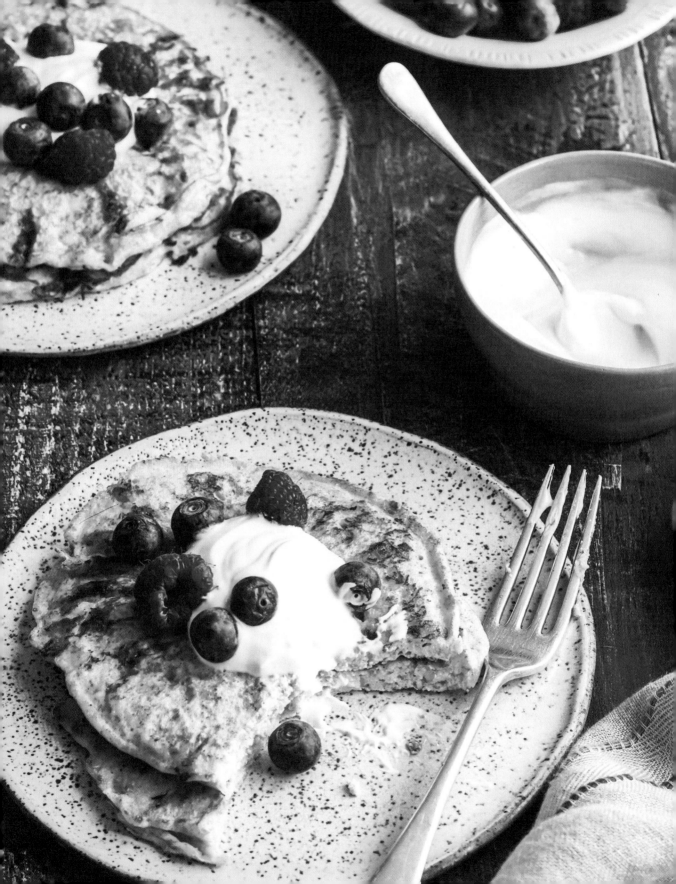

CHAPTER FOUR

Breakfast

Smoothie Bowl with Greek Yogurt and Fresh Berries

MAKES 1 SERVINGS / PREP TIME: 5 MINUTES / COOK TIME: 5 MINUTES
TOTAL TIME: 10 MINUTES

The appearance of our food and where we eat our meals can strongly affect our feelings of satiety after eating. In fact, after surgery, whether you're eating in a high-stress environment or having a relaxing candlelit dinner can influence whether a food makes you sick. Instead of slamming a protein shake for your next breakfast on the way out the door, try sitting down to enjoy this refreshing smoothie bowl. It is just as appealing to the eye as the stomach. Slow down and savor every bite of this smoothie you can eat with a spoon!

¾ cup unsweetened vanilla almond milk or low-fat milk

¼ cup low-fat plain Greek yogurt

⅓ cup (1 handful) fresh spinach

½ scoop (⅛ cup) plain or vanilla protein powder

¼ cup frozen mixed berries

¼ cup fresh raspberries

¼ cup fresh blueberries

1 tablespoon sliced, slivered almonds

1 teaspoon chia seeds

Post-Op Servings

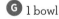 1 bowl

1   In a blender, combine the milk, yogurt, spinach, protein powder, and frozen berries. Blend on high speed for 3 to 4 minutes, until the powder is well dissolved and no longer visible.

2   Pour the smoothie into small bowl.

3   Decorate the smoothie with the fresh raspberries, blueberries, almonds, and chia seeds.

4   Serve with a spoon and enjoy!

Serving tip: *You can make this smoothie bowl with a variety of other fruits and toppings to change it up. Try a mango-pineapple version. Top with unsweetened, flaked coconut and use coconut milk in the smoothie base for a more tropical vibe.*

Per Serving (1 bowl): Calories: 255; Total fat: 10 g; Protein: 20g; Carbs: 21g; Fiber: 8g; Sugar: 10g; Sodium: 262mg

Hearty Slow Cooker Cinnamon Oatmeal

MAKES 10 SERVINGS / PREP TIME: 5 MINUTES / COOK TIME: 7 TO 8 HOURS
TOTAL TIME: 7 TO 8 HOURS

According to the National Weight Control Registry, eating breakfast regularly is a common habit of people who have lost and maintained weight. Unfortunately, it's an easy meal for many to miss. Try this recipe for slow cooker oatmeal to prepare your breakfast the night before and eat throughout the week. And check out the easy tips for increasing the protein content.

8 cups water

2 cups steel-cut oats

2 teaspoons ground cinnamon

1 teaspoon ground nutmeg

Add-ins for protein (per individual serving, limit to 1)

½ cup low-fat milk (add before serving or while reheating)

2 tablespoons unflavored or vanilla protein powder

2 tablespoons nonfat powdered milk or egg white powder

2 tablespoons powdered peanut butter

Add-ins for flavor 8+ weeks post-op (per individual serving, limit to 1)

½ cup fresh or frozen berries

½ apple, pear, peach, or banana, peeled and sliced

¼ cup pumpkin puree

⅛ cup chopped pecans, walnuts, or almonds

1 In a slow cooker, combine the water, oats, cinnamon, and nutmeg. Cover and cook on low for 7 to 8 hours.

2 Choose and mix in one each of your favorite protein and flavor add-ins before serving.

Did You Know? *Oatmeal is loaded with heart-healthy soluble fiber. Diets rich in soluble fiber have been shown to help lower LDL ("bad") cholesterol. Choose oatmeal more often for a quick, filling breakfast and your heart will thank you.*

Per Serving (¾ cup, no add-ins): Calories: 136; Total fat: 2g; Protein: 6g; Carbs: 23g; Fiber: 4g; Sugar: 0g; Sodium: 0mg

Post-Op Servings

P ¼ cup

S ½ cup

G up to ¾ cup

Cherry-Vanilla Baked Oatmeal

MAKES 6 SERVINGS / PREP TIME: 10 MINUTES / COOK TIME: 45 MINUTES
TOTAL TIME: 55 MINUTES

Look no farther than this baked oatmeal recipe to replace your run-of-the-mill coffee shop pastry—the ones that are high in sugar, high in fat, and high in calories. The sweet flavor and hearty ingredients of this baked oatmeal will leave you feeling warm and satisfied on any cold winter morning. Bake for Sunday breakfast and eat leftovers throughout the week.

Nonstick cooking spray
1 cup old-fashioned oats
½ teaspoon ground cinnamon
¾ teaspoon baking powder
1 tablespoon ground flaxseed
3 eggs
1 cup low-fat milk
½ cup low-fat plain Greek yogurt
1 teaspoon vanilla extract
1 teaspoon liquid stevia (optional; to improve sweetness)
1 cup fresh pitted cherries
1 apple, peeled, cored and chopped

Post-Op Servings

Ⓖ ½ cup baked oatmeal (recipe)

1 Preheat the oven to 375°F. Lightly coat an 8-by-8-inch baking dish with the cooking spray.

2 Mix together the oats, cinnamon, baking powder, and flaxseed in a medium bowl. In a separate large bowl, gently whisk the eggs, milk, yogurt, vanilla, and stevia (if using).

3 Add the dry ingredients to the wet and stir to combine. Gently fold in the cherries and apples.

4 Bake for 45 minutes or until the edges start to pull away from the side of the pan and the oatmeal gently bounces back when touched.

5 Divide leftover oatmeal into airtight glass containers. Refrigerate for up to 1 week for quick and easy breakfast, or freeze.

Serving tip: Experiment with the fixings in your baked oatmeal. I like to make my recipes seasonal. Replace the yogurt with pumpkin puree to add a hint of fall. Try using unsweetened dried cranberries instead of cherries for a holiday twist. Swap out apples and cherries for 2 cups fresh berries in spring for a very berry oatmeal! For the creamiest consistency, I recommend topping with a ¼ cup low-fat milk at serving time.

Per Serving (½ cup): Calories: 149; Total fat: 4g; Protein: 8g; Carbs: 21g; Fiber: 4g; Sugar: 9g; Sodium: 71 mg

High-Protein Pancakes

MAKES 4 PANCAKES / PREP TIME: 5 MINUTES / COOK TIME: 5 MINUTES
TOTAL TIME: 10 MINUTES

Craving some Sunday morning flapjacks without refined carbohydrates and added sugary syrup? Look no farther: Try these high-protein pancakes this weekend. Made with simple ingredients already in your pantry and refrigerator, these hotcakes are sure to be a crowd pleaser.

3 eggs

1 cup low-fat cottage cheese

⅓ cup whole-wheat pastry flour

1½ tablespoons coconut oil, melted

Nonstick cooking spray

Post-Op Servings

Ⓢ ½ pancake

Ⓖ 1 to 2 pancakes

1 In large bowl, lightly whisk the eggs.

2 Whisk in the cottage cheese, flour, and coconut oil just until combined.

3 Heat a large skillet or griddle over medium heat, and lightly coat with the cooking spray.

4 Using a measuring cup, pour ⅓ cup of batter into the skillet for each pancake. Cook for 2 to 3 minutes, or until bubbles appear across the surface of each pancake. Flip over the pancakes and cook for 1 to 2 minutes on the other side, or until golden brown.

5 Serve immediately.

Serving tip: *Top these pancakes with fresh berries and plain yogurt, unsweetened applesauce, or sugar-free syrup. You can even try them with natural peanut butter and bananas on a general diet.*

Per Serving (1 pancake): Calories: 182; Total fat: 10g; Protein: 12g; Carbs: 10g; Fiber: 3g; Sugar: 1g; Sodium: 68mg

Pumpkin Muffins with Walnuts and Zucchini

MAKES 2 DOZEN MUFFINS / PREP TIME: 10 MINUTES / COOK TIME: 25 MINUTES
TOTAL TIME: 35 MINUTES

Most muffins you pick up at your local bakery are packed with loads of sugar, white flour, and plenty of fat. Luckily, it's easy to make your own soft and delicious muffins at home with a few healthy twists. These muffins stay light and moist because they are made with shredded zucchini and pureed pumpkin.

Nonstick cooking spray or baking liners

2 cups old-fashioned oats

1¾ cups whole-wheat pastry flour

¼ cup ground flaxseed

2 tablespoons baking powder

1 teaspoon baking soda

1 teaspoon ground cinnamon

¼ teaspoon ground nutmeg

¼ teaspoon ground ginger

¼ teaspoon ground allspice

2 cups shredded zucchini

1 cup canned pumpkin or fresh pumpkin puree

1 cup low-fat milk

4 eggs, lightly beaten

¼ cup unsweetened applesauce

1 teaspoon liquid stevia

½ cup chopped walnuts

1 Preheat the oven to 375°F. Prepare two muffin tins by coating the cups with the cooking spray, or use baking liners.

2 In large bowl, mix together the oats, flour, flaxseed, baking powder, baking soda, cinnamon, nutmeg, ginger, and allspice.

3 In a separate medium bowl mix together the zucchini, pumpkin, milk, eggs, applesauce, and stevia.

4 Add the wet ingredients to the dry and stir to combine. Gently stir in the walnuts.

5 Fill the cups of the muffin tins about half full with the batter.

6 Bake until the muffins are done, when a toothpick inserted in the center comes out clean, about 25 minutes.

Post-Op Servings

 1 muffin

7 Let the muffins cool for 5 minutes before removing them from the tins. Place on a baking rack to finish cooling.

8 Wrap leftover muffins in plastic wrap and freeze. Reheat frozen muffins in the microwave for about 20 seconds.

Ingredient tip: *Put the shredded zucchini in a colander in the sink and press it with the back of a spoon to drain the moisture; pat dry with paper towels before adding to the bowl.*

Did You Know? *Flaxseed is rich in omega-3s. Omega-3 fats have anti-inflammatory effects in the body and may help promote a healthy brain and healthy heart. Ground flaxseed is also a great source of fiber. It can be mixed into smoothies, cereal, or yogurt. It can also be easily added to baked goods. Swap out ¼ cup of flour for ¼ cup of ground flaxseed in any baking recipe to get more of this nutrient-packed seed into your diet!*

Per Serving (1 muffin): Calories: 128; Total fat: 5g; Protein: 5g; Carbs: 18g; Fiber: 3g; Sugar: 1g; Sodium: 86mg

Hard-Boiled Eggs and Avocado on Toast

MAKES 4 TOASTS / PREP TIME: 10 MINUTES / COOK TIME: 10 MINUTES
TOTAL TIME: 20 MINUTES

A diet staple after a sleeve gastrectomy, eggs are packed with protein, vitamins, and minerals. Eggs are rich in choline, which is essential for brain and liver function. Choose organic free-range eggs when possible, as their yolks contain more heart-healthy omega-3 fats than conventional versions. Hard-boil a dozen eggs at a time and keep them on hand to eat throughout the week.

4 eggs

4 slices sprouted whole-wheat bread, such as Angelic Bakehouse Sprouted Grain

1 medium avocado

1 teaspoon hot sauce

Freshly ground black pepper

Post-Op Servings

 1 toast

1 Bring a large pot of water to a rapid boil over high heat.

2 Carefully add the eggs to the boiling water using a spoon, and set a timer for 10 minutes.

3 Immediately transfer the eggs from the boiling water to a strainer, and run cold water over the eggs to stop the cooking process.

4 Once the eggs are cool enough to handle, peel them and slice lengthwise into fourths.

5 Toast the bread.

6 While the bread toasts, mash the avocado with a fork in a small bowl and mix in the hot sauce.

7 Spread the avocado mash evenly across each toast. Top each toast slice with 4 egg slices and season with the black pepper.

Ingredient tip: *Avocado is rich in healthy fat, but also loaded with calories, so portion control is key. Store the pit with any unused portion of avocado, squeeze a teaspoon of lemon juice over the leftovers, and place in an airtight container or wrap in plastic wrap to prevent browning.*

Per Serving (1 toast): Calories: 191; Total fat: 10g; Protein: 10g; Carbs: 15g; Fiber: 5g; Sugar: 1g; Sodium: 214mg

Wisconsin Scrambler with Aged Cheddar Cheese

MAKES 6 SERVINGS / PREP TIME: 10 MINUTES / COOK TIME: 10 MINUTES
TOTAL TIME: 20 MINUTES

In the "Dairy State," many local diners are known for rich breakfasts of eggs cooked in butter, topped with cheese, and served with a side of bacon. Lean up the traditional Wisconsin scrambler recipe by skipping the butter and using lean turkey sausage. Choosing an aged Cheddar cheese instead of a milder version gives more flavor (the older the Cheddar, the sharper the flavor), so you can use a smaller portion and limit the amount of saturated fat.

Nonstick cooking spray

8 ounces extra-lean turkey sausage (nitrate-free)

6 large eggs, beaten

¼ cup fat-free milk

½ teaspoon onion powder

½ teaspoon garlic powder

3 ounces extra-sharp Wisconsin Cheddar cheese, shredded

Post-Op Servings

Ⓢ ½ cup

Ⓖ ½ to 1 cup

1 Coat a large skillet with the cooking spray and place it over medium-high heat. Add the turkey sausage and brown it, using a wooden spoon to break it into small pieces, until cooked through and no longer pink, about 7 minutes.

2 In a medium bowl, whisk together the eggs and milk. Mix in the onion and garlic powders.

3 Add the eggs to the skillet. Reduce the heat to medium-low and stir gently and constantly with a rubber spatula for 5 minutes, until the eggs are fluffy and cooked through.

4 Top with the cheese and serve.

Serving tip: *One of the best tips a colleague has ever given me is to "only eat cheese if you can taste the flavor." Limit cheese intake to recipes where you can savor the flavor, such as crumbling blue cheese on a salad, jazzing up vegetables with Parmigiano-Reggiano, or including a high-protein snack of sliced Gouda with fruit.*

Per Serving (½ cup): Calories: 169; Total fat: 11g; Protein: 15g; Carbs: 2g; Fiber: 0g; Sugar: 1g; Sodium: 413mg

Andrea's Hangry Eggs with Cauliflower

MAKES 2 SERVINGS / PREP TIME: 5 MINUTES / COOK TIME: 5 MINUTES
TOTAL TIME: 10 MINUTES

Hangry: that feeling of being so hungry that you turn angry—and the worst part is that it usually ends in overeating something you didn't want to eat in the first place. To get through a long morning at work, make sure to have a protein-packed breakfast, and pass on sugary cereals and granola bars, which only leave you hangry in an hour. Here is a simple breakfast idea to prevent mid-morning hanger!

½ (10-ounce) bag of frozen cauliflower florets

4 thin slices (nitrate-free) deli ham

Nonstick cooking spray

2 large eggs

Post-Op Servings

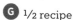 ½ recipe

1 Place the cauliflower with 2 tablespoons water in a microwave-safe bowl or steamer. Cover and cook on high for 4 minutes, or until tender. During the last 30 seconds, add the ham to thoroughly heat it. Drain off any water after cooking.

2 Coat a small skillet with the cooking spray and place it over medium-high heat. Crack two eggs into a small dish and set aside.

3 When the skillet is hot, carefully add the eggs. Reduce the heat to medium-low. Jiggle the pan slightly and then allow eggs to cook for 2 to 3 minutes, or until the whites turn opaque and the yolk starts to cook but is still soft in the center. If necessary, use a rubber spatula to adjust the egg slightly to prevent it from sticking. Place the cauliflower on a plate and the ham on top of the cauliflower. Add the eggs, allowing the yolk to spill over the entire dish. Eat immediately.

Serving tip: *If tolerated, this is also excellent served over steamed asparagus tips instead of cauliflower.*

Per Serving (½ recipe): Calories: 109; Total fat: 6g; Protein: 11g; Carbs: 4g; Fiber: 2g; Sugar: 1g; Sodium: 378mg

Southwestern Scrambled Egg Burritos

MAKES 8 BURRITOS / PREP TIME: 10 MINUTES / COOK TIME: 10 MINUTES
TOTAL TIME: 20 MINUTES

These breakfast burritos have the ingredients you crave but without all the added sodium and fat. Make ahead of time and freeze them, and then toss one in the microwave for a hot breakfast in minutes.

12 eggs

¼ cup low-fat milk

1 teaspoon extra-virgin olive oil

½ onion, chopped

1 red bell pepper, diced

1 green bell pepper, diced

1 (15-ounce) can black beans, drained and rinsed

8 (7- to 8-inch) whole-wheat tortillas, such as La Tortilla Factory low-carb tortillas

1 cup salsa, for serving

Post-Op Servings

S Burrito filling (no tortilla)

G ½ to 1 burrito

1 In a large bowl, whisk together the eggs and milk. Set aside.

2 In a large skillet over medium-high heat, heat the olive oil and add the onion and bell peppers. Sauté for 2 to 3 minutes, or until tender. Add the beans and stir to combine.

3 Add the egg mixture. Reduce the heat to medium-low and stir gently and constantly with a rubber spatula for 5 minutes, until the eggs are fluffy and cooked through.

4 Divide the scrambled egg mixture among the tortillas. Fold over the bottom end of the tortilla, fold in the sides, and roll tightly to close.

5 Serve immediately with the salsa, or place each burrito in a zip-top bag and refrigerate for up to 1 week. To eat, reheat each burrito in the microwave for 60 to 90 seconds. These will also keep well in the freezer for up to 1 month.

Serving tip: *To get more vegetables into your breakfast, buy a bag of frozen California-blend mixed vegetables. Heat some in a skillet with extra-virgin olive oil, add eggs, and—voilà!—a quick veggie-packed egg burrito.*

Per Serving (1 burrito): Calories: 250; Total fat: 10g; Protein: 19g; Carbs: 28g; Fiber: 13g; Sugar: 1g; Sodium: 546mg

Farmer's Egg Casserole with Broccoli, Mushroom, and Onions

SERVES 12 / PREP TIME: 10 MINUTES / COOK TIME: 40 MINUTES
TOTAL TIME: 50 MINUTES

Just because you're on a new diet post-operatively doesn't mean it has to be boring or not flavorful. And it doesn't mean you can't serve it to family and guests. After all, they like healthy, flavorful food as much as the next person. This egg casserole feeds a crowd, and you can put it together the night before. It's also a great way to use up leftover roasted turkey or chicken from last night's dinner.

Nonstick cooking spray

2 teaspoons extra-virgin olive oil

1 onion, diced

½ cup chopped mushrooms

2 cups roughly chopped broccoli florets

12 eggs

2 tablespoons low-fat milk

½ teaspoon dried oregano

½ teaspoon dried basil

¼ teaspoon dried thyme

1 cup chopped or shredded cooked poultry breast, such as leftover turkey or chicken, canned chicken breast, or turkey lunch meat (nitrate-free)

1 cup shredded Swiss cheese

¼ cup shredded Parmigiano-Reggiano cheese

1 Preheat the oven to 350°F. Spray a 9-by-13-inch baking dish with the cooking spray.

2 In a large skillet over medium heat, add the olive oil. When the oil is hot, add the onion and sauté for 1 to 2 minutes, or until tender. Add the mushrooms and cook for an additional 2 to 3 minutes, or until tender.

3 In a steamer or microwave-safe bowl, place the broccoli florets and 2 tablespoons water. Cover and microwave/steam for about 4 minutes or just until tender. Drain off any liquid and set aside.

4 In a large bowl, whisk together the eggs, milk, oregano, basil, and thyme.

5 Add the cooked vegetables, poultry, and Swiss cheese to the egg mixture and stir to combine.

6 Pour the mixture into the baking dish and sprinkle the Parmigiano-Reggiano cheese over the top.

Post-Op Servings

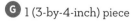 1 (3-by-4-inch) piece

7 Bake for 35 to 40 minutes, or until lightly browned. Let the casserole rest for 5 minutes before serving.

8 Store leftovers in the refrigerator for up to 1 week. Reheat before eating.

Serving tip: *Customize this egg casserole with whatever is in your pantry. Try to use vegetables that are in season. Try a Southwest version with chopped bell peppers and topped with fresh salsa. Make a spinach-artichoke bake with canned artichoke hearts. Egg casseroles can be a great way to get plenty of vegetables and a variety of proteins, so shake it up to keep it interesting.*

Per Serving (1 [3-by-4-inch] piece): Calories: 147; Total fat: 10g; Protein: 12g; Carbs: 2g; Fiber: 1g; Sugar: 0g; Sodium: 193mg

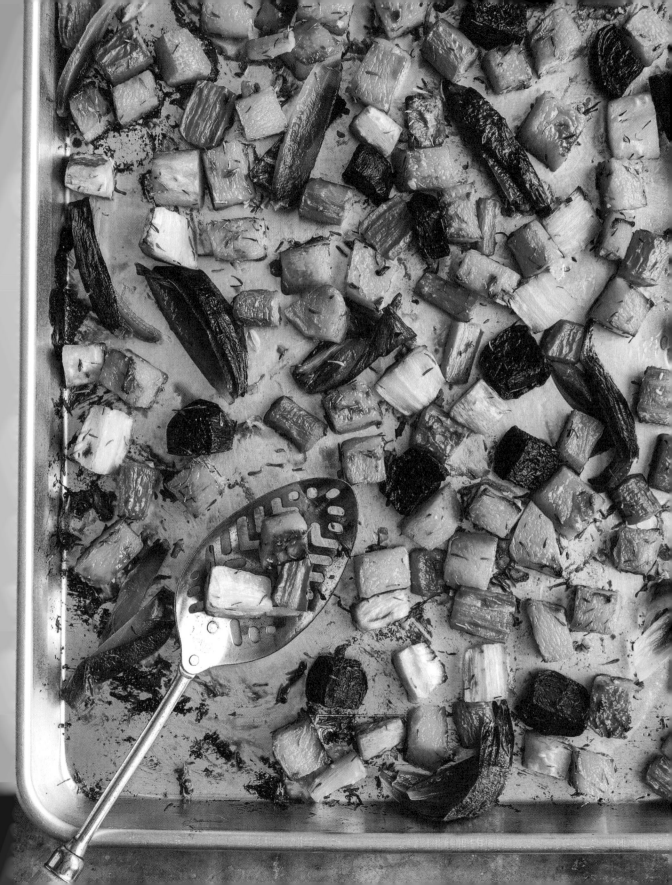

CHAPTER FIVE

Sides and Snacks

Mashed Cauliflower

MAKES 3 CUPS / PREP TIME: 10 MINUTES / COOK TIME: 5 MINUTES
TOTAL TIME: 15 MINUTES

Potatoes are a staple of the American diet and a side dish on many a dinner plate. Unfortunately, when we take these starchy spuds and deep-fry them or load them with butter and sour cream, we surpass our daily allowance for carbohydrates, fat, and calories. Try swapping your traditional spuds for this twist on mashed potatoes. You will save on calories and carbohydrates yet still feel comforted by the creamy nature of this simple dish.

1 large head cauliflower

¼ cup water

⅓ cup low-fat buttermilk

1 tablespoon minced garlic

1 tablespoon extra-virgin olive oil

Post-Op Servings

P ¼ cup

S ½ cup

G ½ cup

1 Break the cauliflower into small florets. Place in a large microwave-safe bowl with the water. Cover and microwave for about 5 minutes, or until the cauliflower is soft. Drain the water from the bowl.

2 In a blender or food processor, puree the buttermilk, cauliflower, garlic, and olive oil on medium speed until the cauliflower is smooth and creamy.

3 Serve immediately.

Ingredient tip: *You can buy buttermilk in most supermarkets, but it's just as easy to make your own. Mix 1 teaspoon freshly squeezed lemon juice with ⅓ cup low-fat milk. Let the mixture sit for about 10 minutes, or until the milk begins to thicken.*

Cooking tip: *For even more flavor, microwave the cauliflower with chicken or vegetable broth instead of water and add ½ cup shredded Parmigiano-Reggiano cheese when you puree the mixture. You can add protein to this dish by blending in powdered egg whites or unflavored protein powder after the first puree (puree until smooth and creamy; then add the protein powder and puree to incorporate).*

Per Serving (½ cup): Calories: 62; Total fat: 2g; Protein: 3g; Carbs: 8g; Fiber: 3g; Sugar: 3g; Sodium: 54mg

Simple Spinach Dip

MAKES 12 SERVINGS / PREP TIME: 10 MINUTES, PLUS 2 HOURS TO CHILL
TOTAL TIME: 2 HOURS, 10 MINUTES

It's certainly easy to max out on fat and calories after only a few bites of traditional spinach dip. And who can stop after only a few bites of this rich, creamy appetizer? Save on calories without compromising flavor with this simple spinach dip recipe that uses Greek yogurt instead of sour cream. Use whole seasonings and herbs instead of a premixed packet to cut back on sodium, leave out the MSG, and improve the flavor.

1 cup plain nonfat Greek yogurt

4 ounces Neufchâtel cheese

½ cup olive oil-based mayonnaise

2 teaspoons minced garlic

1½ teaspoons onion powder

1 teaspoon smoked paprika

¾ teaspoon freshly ground black pepper

¼ teaspoon red pepper flakes

2 teaspoons Worcestershire sauce

1 (8-ounce) can water chestnuts, drained and finely chopped

½ cup chopped scallions

1 (10-ounce) package frozen chopped spinach, thawed and squeezed of excess moisture

1 In a large bowl, use a hand mixer on low speed to mix the yogurt, Neufchâtel cheese, mayonnaise, garlic, onion powder, paprika, black pepper, red pepper flakes, and Worcestershire sauce.

2 Add the water chestnuts, scallions, and spinach and stir by hand until well combined.

3 Cover and refrigerate for at least 2 hours prior to serving, or overnight.

4 Serve with raw vegetables or whole-grain crackers.

Serving tip: *Use as a spread on deli-sliced (nitrate-free) turkey and roll it up for a quick snack or a simple lunch. Or substitute for mayo or mustard on an open-face sandwich. The possibilities abound.*

Per Serving (¼ cup): Calories: 71; Total fat: 4g; Protein: 3g; Carbs: 5g; Fiber: 1g; Sugar: 2g; Sodium: 131 mg

Post-Op Servings

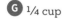 ¼ cup

Pickle Roll-Ups

MAKES ABOUT 40 MINI ROLL-UPS / PREP TIME: 20 MINUTES
TOTAL TIME: 20 MINUTES

Pickles have a crisp, sour, delicious taste and almost no calories. Here is an easy recipe to make as a low-carb appetizer for your next family gathering or just for a simple snack. You can even pack them for your lunch when you're in a hurry. The pickles will satisfy your craving to "crunch" without all the added calories.

¼ pound deli ham (nitrate-free), thinly sliced (about 8 slices)

8 ounces Neufchâtel cheese, at room temperature

1 teaspoon dried dill

1 teaspoon onion powder

8 whole kosher dill pickle spears

Post-Op Servings

G 5 roll-ups (1 entire pickle roll-up)

1 Get a large cutting board or clean counter space to assemble your roll-ups.

2 Lay the ham slices on the work surface and carefully spread on the Neufchâtel cheese.

3 Season each lightly with the dill and onion powder.

4 Place an entire pickle on an end of the ham and carefully roll.

5 Slice each pickle roll-up into mini rounds about ½- to 1-inch wide.

6 Skew each with a toothpick for easier serving.

Did You Know? *There is any number of foods with gut-healthy probiotics. Yogurt, fresh sauerkraut, and—you guessed it—pickles contain beneficial bacteria that keep your gastrointestinal tract regular and may even be linked to healthy body weight.*

Per Serving (1 roll-up): Calories: 86; Total fat: 7g; Protein: 4g; Carbs: 4g; Fiber: 0 g; Sugar: 2g; Sodium: 540mg

Baked Zucchini Fries

MAKES 6 SERVINGS / PREP TIME: 15 MINUTES / COOK TIME: 30 MINUTES
TOTAL TIME: 45 MINUTES

The salty taste of french fries is a comfort to many people—and fries are one of those foods that you can't eat just one of. After the gastric sleeve, fried food is off limits—not only because it's loaded with fat and calories, but also because it can make you feel sick. But there are plenty of healthier "fries" out there that can sate any cravings. These zucchini fries are the perfect substitute. So enjoy your next side of fries—guilt free!

3 large zucchini

2 large eggs

1 cup whole-wheat
    bread crumbs

¼ cup shredded
    Parmigiano-
    Reggiano cheese

1 teaspoon garlic powder

1 teaspoon onion powder

Post-Op Servings

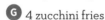 4 zucchini fries

1 Preheat the oven to 425°F. Line a large rimmed baking sheet with aluminum foil.

2 Halve each zucchini lengthwise and continue slicing each piece into fries about ½ inch in diameter. You will have about 8 strips per zucchini.

3 In a small bowl, crack the eggs and beat lightly.

4 In a medium bowl, combine the bread crumbs, Parmigiano-Reggiano cheese, garlic powder, and onion powder.

5 One by one, dip each zucchini strip into the egg, then roll it in the bread crumb mixture. Place on the prepared baking sheet.

6 Roast for 30 minutes, stirring the fries halfway through. Zucchini fries are done when brown and crispy.

7 Serve immediately.

Per Serving (4 fries): Calories: 89; Total fat: 3g; Protein: 5g; Carbs: 10g; Fiber: 1g; Sugar: 3g; Sodium: 179mg

Italian Eggplant Pizzas

MAKES 6 SERVINGS / PREP TIME: 15 MINUTES / COOK TIME: 30 MINUTES
TOTAL TIME: 45 MINUTES

These mini pizzas are great as an appetizer or snack, or can serve as a meal by themselves—especially if you are looking for some variety when on the soft diet. Plus, it's a great way to include eggplant in your diet, a vegetable rich in potassium and fiber yet often overlooked at the farmers' market or grocery store. Mix up your toppings and even the cheese you use to create some variety on these mini low-carb pizzas.

1 large eggplant, cut into ¼- to ½-inch rounds

1 tablespoon salt

1 tablespoon extra-virgin olive oil

2 teaspoons minced garlic

½ teaspoon dried oregano

1 cup Marinara Sauce with Italian Herbs (page 178)

1 cup fresh basil leaves

1 cup shredded part-skim Mozzarella cheese

¼ cup shredded Parmigiano-Reggiano cheese

Post-Op Servings

S 1 to 2 eggplant pizza rounds

G 2 to 4 eggplant pizza rounds

1 Preheat the oven to 425°F. Line a large rimmed baking sheet with aluminum foil.

2 Put the eggplant rounds on paper towels and sprinkle them with the salt. Let them sit for 10 to 15 minutes to help release some of the water in the eggplant. Pat dry afterward. It's okay to wipe off some of the salt before baking.

3 In a small bowl, mix together the olive oil, garlic, and oregano.

4 Place the eggplant rounds 1-inch apart on the baking sheet. Using a pastry brush, coat each side of the eggplant with the olive oil mixture. Bake the eggplant for 15 minutes.

5 Create pizzas by layering 1 to 2 tablespoons of marinara sauce, 2 basil leaves, about 1 tablespoon of mozzarella cheese, and about ½ tablespoon of Parmigiano-Reggiano cheese on each baked eggplant round.

6 Bake the pizzas for an additional 10 minutes or until the cheese is melted and starting to brown.

7 Serve immediately and enjoy!

Per Serving (2 eggplant pizza rounds): Calories: 99; Total fat: 6g; Protein: 5g; Carbs: 7g; Fiber: 2g; Sugar: 4g; Sodium: 500mg

Tomato, Basil, and Cucumber Salad

MAKES 4 SERVINGS / PREP TIME: 15 MINUTES, PLUS 30 MINUTES TO CHILL
TOTAL TIME: 45 MINUTES

One of the most delicious parts about summertime is enjoying a refreshing salad—especially if you can make it with fresh produce from the farmers' market or your garden. The flavors and nutrients of fresh, in-season vegetables are like nothing else. This is an easy salad to make and it will complement any meal—and since it's lettuce-free, it's a great way to get out of your usual salad rut.

1 large cucumber, seeded and sliced

4 medium tomatoes, quartered

1 medium red onion, thinly sliced

½ cup chopped fresh basil

3 tablespoons red wine vinegar

1 tablespoon extra-virgin olive oil

½ teaspoon Dijon mustard

½ teaspoon freshly ground black pepper

Post-Op Servings

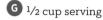 G 1/2 cup serving

1 In a medium bowl, mix together the cucumber, tomatoes, red onion, and basil.

2 In a small bowl, whisk together the vinegar, olive oil, mustard, and pepper.

3 Pour the dressing over the vegetables, and gently stir until well combined.

4 Cover and chill for at least 30 minutes prior to serving.

Serving tip: *Turn this salad into a well-rounded meal by grilling up some chicken breast and cutting it into 1-inch pieces. Gently toss the chicken in the salad for a refreshing and filling lunch or dinner.*

Per Serving (½ cup): Calories: 72; Total fat: 4g; Protein: 1g; Carbs: 8g; Fiber: 1g; Sugar: 4g; Sodium: 5mg

Black Bean Chipotle Hummus

MAKES ABOUT 1½ CUPS / PREP TIME: 5 MINUTES / COOK TIME: 5 MINUTES
TOTAL TIME: 10 MINUTES

We usually don't think about the condiments we add to our food. A little catsup here, a dab of butter or mayo there, or a little drizzle of ranch dressing over the salad. The flavor addition is great—the excess calories and fat, far less so. Try using hummus as an alternative spread on top of burgers, rolled in lunch meat, or as a dip for raw vegetables. Standard hummus is made with chickpeas, tahini, olive oil, and lemon juice—this twist is made with black beans and smoky chipotle flavor.

1 (15.5-ounce) can black beans, drained and rinsed

Juice of 1 lime

1 chipotle pepper in adobo sauce

1 teaspoon adobo sauce

1 teaspoon minced garlic

2 teaspoons ground cumin

2 tablespoons extra-virgin olive oil

¼ cup chopped fresh cilantro

Post-Op Servings

2 tablespoons

1 In a food processor or blender, puree the black beans, lime juice, chipotle pepper, adobo sauce, garlic, cumin, olive oil, and cilantro on high until very smooth, 2 to 3 minutes.

2 If the hummus is very thick, add an additional 1 to 2 tablespoons of water to reach your desired consistency.

3 Serve immediately or store in an airtight container for up to 1 week.

Ingredient tip: *Purchase chipotle peppers in adobo sauce, canned, in the ethnic food aisle of your grocery store. Save extra chipotle peppers in an airtight container and use within 1 week. Try using them in the Slow Cooker Barbecue Shredded Chicken (page 135) or Chipotle Shredded Pork (page 146).*

Per Serving (2 tablespoons): Calories: 52; Total fat: 2g; Protein: 2g; Carbs: 6g; Fiber: 2g; Sugar: 0g; Sodium: 26mg

Roasted Root Vegetables

MAKES ABOUT 6 CUPS / PREP TIME: 15 MINUTES / COOK TIME: 45 MINUTES
TOTAL TIME: 60 MINUTES

This is a great recipe to help you get several servings of vegetables in a variety of colors. Roasting any vegetables in the oven brings out their natural sweet taste and all sorts of other flavors you didn't even know were possible from something so simple. I especially love the combination of these root vegetables—they seem to taste even better the next day. Try these roasted vegetables and you will instantly become a vegetable lover!

Nonstick cooking spray

2 medium red
  beets, peeled

2 large parsnips, peeled

2 large carrots, peeled

1 medium butternut
  squash (about
  2 pounds), peeled
  and seeded

1 medium red onion

2 tablespoons extra-virgin
  olive oil

4 teaspoons minced garlic

2 teaspoons dried thyme

Post-Op Servings

Ⓢ ¼ cup serving

Ⓖ ½ to 1 cup serving

1 Preheat the oven to 425°F. Spray a large rimmed baking sheet with the cooking spray.

2 Roughly chop the beets, parsnips, carrots, and butternut squash into 1-inch pieces. Cut the onion into half and then each half into 4 large chunks.

3 Arrange the vegetables in a single, even layer on the baking sheet, and sprinkle them with the olive oil, garlic, and thyme. Use a spoon to mix the vegetables to coat them with the oil and seasonings.

4 Roast for 45 minutes, stirring the vegetables every 15 minutes, until all the vegetables are tender.

5 Serve immediately.

Cooking tip: *Don't let your vegetables spoil before you can eat them. When you think vegetables might be starting to go bad, clean out your refrigerator drawer and roast them. Use roasted vegetables on a salad, as a side dish, on top of pizza, or puree them into a soup.*

Per Serving (½ cup): Calories: 68; Total fat: 3g; Protein: 1g; Carbs: 11g; Fiber: 1g; Sugar: 5g; Sodium: 30mg

Cauliflower Rice

MAKES 4 CUPS / PREP TIME: 5 MINUTES / COOK TIME: 5 MINUTES
TOTAL TIME: 10 MINUTES

Rice is a staple on the typical dinner table for many meals in the United States and across the world. It's quick and easy to make, but it's also dense in calories and carbohydrates. Swapping traditional white rice for a brown or wild rice improves the health factor (more nutrients and fiber), but these varieties still contain the same amount of calories and carbohydrates. Cut back on starchy foods by using riced cauliflower as a side dish. You will cut calories and carbohydrates by one-eighth!

1 cauliflower head
1 teaspoon extra-virgin
   olive oil

Post-Op Servings

 1/4 cup

1 Prepare the cauliflower head by removing the stems and leaves. Cut it into four large sections.

2 Put the cauliflower in a food processor and pulse until it breaks down into pieces the size of rice. You may need to remove any leftover pieces of stem. Alternatively, you can use a box grater to shred the cauliflower.

3 Transfer the riced cauliflower to a plate or bowl and pat it dry with a paper towel.

4 Place a small skillet over medium heat and add the olive oil. When the oil is hot, add the cauliflower. Sauté for 5 to 6 minutes, or until tender. Alternatively, steam the cauliflower rice and drain off any excess liquid before serving.

Serving tip: *If your family is slow to make the low-carb conversion to cauliflower rice, mix half and half with regular rice. Use riced cauliflower instead of regular rice in stir fries, under baked salmon with vegetables, or in soups or curries.*

Per Serving (¼ cup): Calories: 12; Total fat: 0g; Protein: 1g; Carbs: 2g; Fiber: 1g; Sugar: 1g; Sodium: 5mg

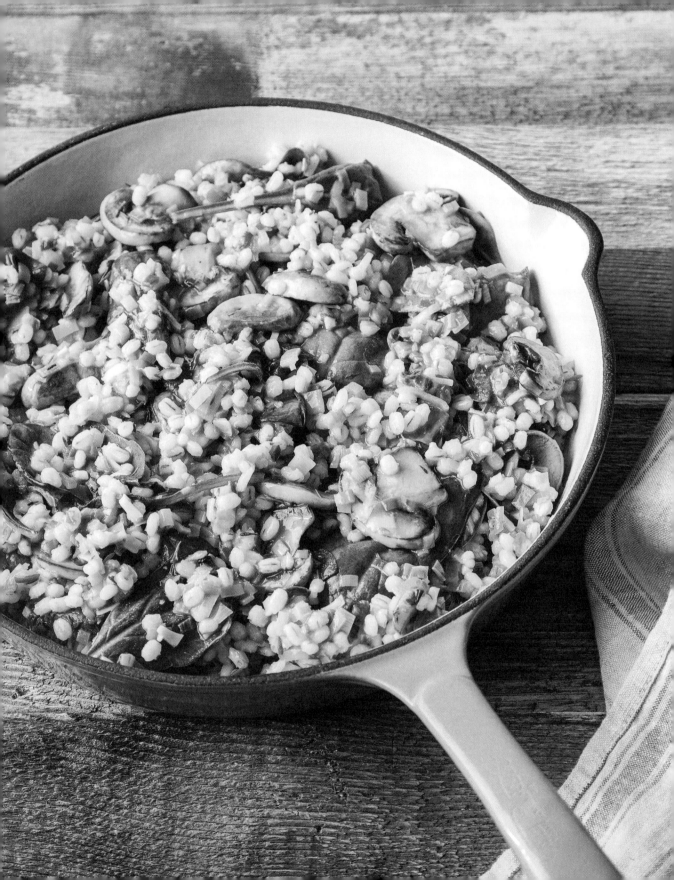

CHAPTER SIX

Vegetarian Dinners

Roasted Vegetable Quinoa Salad with Chickpeas

MAKES 6 SERVINGS / PREP TIME: 15 MINUTES / COOK TIME: 30 MINUTES
TOTAL TIME: 45 MINUTES

Many people find that their sleeve tolerates cooked vegetables better than raw vegetables in the initial months post-op. This quinoa salad is an excellent alternative to traditional lettuce salads. It contains a variety of vegetarian protein sources—quinoa and chickpeas—and it's loaded with vegetables that have been roasted to bring out their natural rich flavors.

1 small eggplant, diced

1 small zucchini, diced

1 small yellow summer squash, diced

½ cup grape tomatoes, halved

1 (15-ounce) can chickpeas, drained and rinsed

3 tablespoons extra-virgin olive oil, divided

⅓ cup packaged quinoa

1 cup low-sodium vegetable or chicken broth

2 tablespoons freshly squeezed lemon juice

1 teaspoon minced fresh garlic or 1 garlic clove, minced

1 tablespoon dried basil

1 teaspoon dried oregano

1 Preheat the oven to 425°F. Line a 9-by-13-inch baking sheet with parchment paper.

2 Spread the eggplant, zucchini, yellow squash, tomatoes, and chickpeas across the baking sheet and toss them with 1 tablespoon of olive oil.

3 Bake for 30 minutes, stirring once halfway through. The finished vegetables should be tender and the tomatoes should be juicy. The chickpeas will be firm and crispy.

4 While the vegetables and chickpeas are roasting, place the quinoa and broth in a small saucepan over medium-high heat. Cover and bring to a boil. Reduce the heat to low and cook for about 15 minutes, or until all liquid has absorbed. Remove the pan from the heat and fluff the quinoa with a fork. (Otherwise, make the quinoa according to the package instructions.)

Post-Op Servings

½ cup serving

5　In a small dish, whisk together the lemon juice, garlic, and remaining 2 tablespoons of olive oil. Mix in the basil and oregano.

6　In a large serving bowl, combine the quinoa, roasted vegetables with chickpeas, and dressing. Gently stir to combine. Serve and enjoy!

Serving tip: *To increase the protein in this dish, you can add lean grilled chicken breast or serve with a piece of baked fish. You can always top with a dollop of low-fat plain Greek yogurt.*

Per Serving (½ cup): Calories: 200; Total fat: 9g; Protein: 7g; Carbs: 27g; Fiber: 8g; Sugar: 4g; Sodium: 160mg

Mexican Stuffed Summer Squash

MAKES 2 SERVINGS / PREP TIME: 5 MINUTES / COOK TIME: 33 MINUTES
TOTAL TIME: 38 MINUTES

Here is a great low-carb dish that will satisfy your cravings and use some of summer's most plentiful vegetables. It's easy enough to double or triple to make for a family or for you to eat throughout the week.

Nonstick cooking spray

1 yellow summer squash

½ cup Refried Black Beans (page 58) or canned fat-free refried pinto beans with 1 teaspoon taco seasoning mixed in (for flavor)

½ cup cooked quinoa

¼ cup shredded Colby Jack cheese

1 small tomato, diced

2 tablespoons sliced black olives

2 scallions, chopped, for garnish

Post-Op Servings

G 1 stuffed squash half

1 Preheat the oven to 400°F. Coat an 8-by-8-inch baking dish with the cooking spray.

2 Cut the ends off of the summer squash and discard. Cut lengthwise, then use a spoon to remove and discard the seeds. Place the squash halves cut-side down in the baking dish. Gently poke a couple of holes in the squash to vent. Add 1 tablespoon of water to the dish. Microwave for about 3 minutes or until slightly tender. Discard any leftover water.

3 When cool enough to handle, turn the squash so they are skin-side down and spaced evenly apart in the dish.

4 Layer ¼ cup of the beans in each squash, then ¼ cup of the quinoa. Top the whole thing with the Colby Jack cheese. Cover with aluminum foil and bake for 25 minutes. Remove the foil and bake for 5 minutes more, or until the cheese is bubbly and the squash is tender.

5 Garnish each squash with the tomatoes, olives, and scallions just before serving.

Serving tip: *Get creative with extras. Brown ground turkey or a soy-based meat substitute in taco seasoning and add on top of the beans. Sauté bell peppers and onions to layer on or serve with avocado and cilantro.*

Per Serving (1 squash half): Calories: 190; Total fat: 8 g; Protein: 9g; Carbs: 21g; Fiber: 4g; Sugar: 3g; Sodium: 40mg

Cheesy Broccoli Soup

MAKES 8 SERVINGS / PREP TIME: 10 MINUTES / COOK TIME: 20 MINUTES
TOTAL TIME: 30 MINUTES

Who doesn't love Panera Bread's Broccoli Cheddar soup? It's so rich, creamy, and satisfying. Knowing these are the types of meals my patients craved in the months after bariatric surgery, I set out to create my own version that offers all the flavor and texture of the soup with far fewer calories and less fat. I hope this recipe will have your taste buds and your family fooled!

1 tablespoon extra-virgin olive oil

1 medium onion, chopped

1 tablespoon minced garlic

2 cups grated carrots

¼ teaspoon ground nutmeg

¼ cup whole-wheat pastry flour

2 cups low-sodium vegetable broth

2 cups nonfat or 1% milk

½ cup fat-free half-and-half

3 cups broccoli florets

2 cups shredded extra-sharp Cheddar cheese

Post-Op Servings

P ¼ cup

S ½ cup

G 1 to 2 cups

1 In a stock pot, heat the olive oil over medium heat. Add the onion and garlic. Stir until fragrant, about 1 minute. Add the carrots and continue to stir until tender, about 2 to 3 minutes.

2 Add the nutmeg and the flour. Continue to cook, stirring constantly, until browned, 2 to 3 minutes. Add the broth and then the milk, and whisk constantly until it starts to thicken. Add the half-and-half and mix to combine well.

3 Stir in the broccoli florets. Bring to a boil and then reduce the heat to a simmer. Cook for 10 minutes or until the broccoli is tender. Use an immersion blender to puree it to a smooth consistency, if desired, or leave it as is for a chunky soup.

4 Stir in the Cheddar cheese until melted. Reserve some cheese as a topping for serving time.

5 Refrigerate any leftovers and eat within 1 week.

Per Serving (1 cup): Calories: 193; Total fat: 9g; Protein: 12g; Carbs: 17g; Fiber: 4g; Sugar: 7g; Sodium: 450mg

Red Lentil Soup with Kale

MAKES 6 SERVINGS / PREP TIME: 10 MINUTES / COOK TIME: 45 MINUTES
TOTAL TIME: 55 MINUTES

Eating vegetarian can be just as filling as eating a diet high in animal protein when you choose the right foods. Warm up with this hearty lentil soup—loaded with filling fiber and flavorful herbs and seasonings. Keep a bag of lentils on hand so you can whip up this hearty soup on the next cold winter night.

1 tablespoon extra-virgin olive oil

1 cup chopped onion

½ cup carrots, cut into ½-inch chunks

½ cup celery, cut into ¼-inch chunks

1 teaspoon minced garlic

1 cup red lentils

1 teaspoon dried thyme

1 teaspoon ground cumin

2 cups low-sodium vegetable broth

2 cups water

2 large stalks kale, stemmed, with leaves chopped (about 2 cups)

1 bay leaf

2 tablespoons freshly squeezed lemon juice

Low-fat plain Greek yogurt (optional)

Post-Op Servings

P ¼ cup

S ½ cup

G 1 to 2 cups

1 In a large stock pot over medium heat, heat the olive oil. Add the onion, carrots, celery, and garlic, and sauté until tender, 5 to 7 minutes.

2 Add the lentils, thyme, and cumin. Mix well and stir for 1 to 2 minutes, until all the ingredients are coated well with the seasonings.

3 Add the broth and water to the pot. Bring to a simmer, add the kale, and stir well. Add the bay leaf, then cover the pot and simmer for 30 to 35 minutes.

4 Remove the pot from the heat. Remove and discard the bay leaf. Stir in the lemon juice. Use an immersion blender to puree the soup to your desired consistency. Alternatively, let the soup cool for 10 minutes before pureeing it in batches in a blender.

5 Garnish each bowl of soup with a dollop of the Greek yogurt (if using) and serve.

Post-op tip: *If you're cooking this during the post-op pureed stage, add 1 to 2 tablespoons of egg white powder or unflavored protein powder after cooking to increase the protein content.*

Per Serving (1 cup): Calories: 170; Total fat: 3g; Protein: 13g; Carbs: 24g; Fiber: 3g; Sugar: 4g; Sodium: 59mg

Barley-Mushroom Risotto

MAKES 6 SERVINGS / PREP TIME: 5 MINUTES / COOK TIME: 55 MINUTES
TOTAL TIME: 60 MINUTES

I love the flavor and concept of risotto, but I'm always looking for a healthier alternative. Barley is a nutrient-packed grain (found at a bargain price, I might add!) that you can use to replace the Arborio rice in risotto. Barley is higher in fiber, especially soluble fiber, which has been shown to lower LDL ("bad") cholesterol. I also love how this risotto dish is loaded with mushrooms and spinach to sneak in some vegetables while still maximizing flavor.

1 tablespoon extra-virgin olive oil

1 teaspoon minced garlic

2 leeks, cleaned, ends removed and finely chopped, both white and green parts

4 cups sliced mushrooms

2 teaspoons dried thyme

½ cup pearl barley

½ cup dry white wine

1½ cups low-sodium vegetable or chicken broth

1 cup water

3 cups fresh spinach leaves

Post-Op Servings

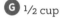 G ½ cup

1 Place a large skillet over medium heat. Sauté the olive oil and garlic for 1 minute. Add the leeks and sauté for 2 to 3 minutes, or until tender.

2 Add the mushrooms and cook until tender and browned, about 4 minutes.

3 Stir in the thyme and barley. Cook for another 2 minutes.

4 Add the wine and stir. Simmer for about 5 minutes, or until the liquid is absorbed.

5 Add the broth and water. Reduce the heat to low, cover the skillet, and simmer for 40 minutes. Stir occasionally to make sure the barley does not stick to the bottom of the pan.

6 Gently stir in the spinach and mix until it is wilted. Serve immediately.

Serving tip: *Although barley is higher in protein than rice, this dish isn't particularly protein-loaded. Add some Parmigiano-Reggiano cheese, roasted tofu, or serve on the side of a chicken breast or lean pork chop to help you meet your protein goal for the day.*

Per Serving (½ cup): Calories: 104; Total fat: 3g; Protein: 3g; Carbs: 16g; Fiber: 3g; Sugar: 1g; Sodium: 40mg

Coconut Curry Tofu Bowl

MAKES 6 SERVINGS / PREP TIME: 15 MINUTES, PLUS 30 MINUTES TO DRAIN
COOK TIME: 30 MINUTES / TOTAL TIME: 1 HOUR, 15 MINUTES

Adding some seasoning with herbs and spices and experimenting with vegetarian proteins are both great ways to shake up what can seem like a monotonous rotation of protein shakes, steamed vegetables, and baked fish. Tofu is a great substitute for meat—it's heart-healthy, loaded with protein, and inexpensive. It soaks up the flavor of all the seasonings it's cooked in. When you use the extra-firm variety and sauté it, it even has the same texture as meat. Don't skip over a recipe just because it has a long list of ingredients. Most likely, many of them are pantry items you already have on hand. Buying frozen minced garlic and freezing fresh ginger root means you always have them on hand.

1 (14-ounce) package extra-firm tofu

3 teaspoons coconut oil, divided

4 teaspoons minced garlic

1 tablespoon grated ginger

1 jalapeño pepper, seeds removed and finely diced

1 yellow or orange bell pepper, chopped

2 carrots, cut into ½-inch chunks

1 medium bok choy, stems cut into ½-inch pieces, leaves diced

2 tablespoons curry powder

½ teaspoon turmeric

½ teaspoon ground cumin

⅛ teaspoon ground cinnamon

1 Drain the tofu and place it on a paper towel–lined plate or bowl. Cover with several layers of paper towel or a clean dish towel, and set a sauté pan on top for added weight. Let the tofu sit for 30 minutes to drain some of its excess water.

2 Place the tofu on a clean cutting board. Halve it lengthwise, and then cut into 1-by-2-inch cubes.

3 In a large nonstick pan over medium heat, heat 1½ teaspoons of coconut oil.

4 When the oil is very hot, add the tofu cubes and cook until lightly browned on all sides, 10 to 15 minutes. Transfer the tofu to a bowl and set aside.

5 In the same pan over medium heat, add the remaining 1½ teaspoons of coconut oil. Once the oil is very hot, add the garlic, ginger, jalapeño, bell pepper, carrots, and bok choy stems. Sauté for 10 minutes, or until the vegetables are crisp tender.

2 cups unflavored, unsweetened coconut milk

4 ounces canned tomato sauce

½ cup low-sodium vegetable or chicken broth

Cauliflower Rice (page 85)

¼ cup chopped fresh cilantro, for garnish

Post-Op Servings

G ½ to 1 cup serving

6 Add the curry powder, turmeric, cumin, and cinnamon and stir to coat.

7 Next, mix in the coconut milk, tomato sauce, and broth. Stir until smooth.

8 Gently mix in the tofu and bok choy leaves. Stir to coat and allow to simmer for 5 to 10 minutes, or until the leaves are wilted.

9 Prepare the bowls by layering the Cauliflower Rice and curry tofu vegetable mixture. Garnish each bowl with the cilantro.

Cooking tip: *Use this recipe as a base and change up the vegetables. Add butternut squash; use kale or spinach instead of bok choy; swap sweet potatoes for the carrots. Choose in-season vegetables when possible. This recipe also works well with frozen veggies.*

Per Serving (1 cup): Calories: 219; Total fat: 8g; Protein: 15g; Carbs: 24g; Fiber: 11g; Sugar: 10g; Sodium: 337mg

Eggplant Rollatini

MAKES 6 TO 8 ROLLATINI / PREP TIME: 15 MINUTES / COOK TIME: 50 MINUTES
TOTAL TIME: 1 HOUR, 5 MINUTES

Italian food is warm and comforting, yet it's often loaded with greasy beef or sausage and served with carb-laden noodles. Even vegetarian options like eggplant parmagiana still tend to be deep-fried and carb heavy. This recipe has all the flavor of a wholesome Italian dinner without the carbs and the fat. The best part is you can still eat the ooey-gooey cheese but with far fewer calories and fat than you would have with most traditional dishes.

Nonstick cooking spray

1 large eggplant

1 tablespoon salt

1 teaspoon extra-virgin olive oil

1 pound fresh spinach (about 10 cups)

½ cup part-skim ricotta cheese

¾ cup shredded part-skim mozzarella cheese, divided

¼ cup shredded Parmigiano-Reggiano cheese

1 egg

1 teaspoon minced garlic

½ cup Marinara Sauce with Italian Herbs (page 178) or low-sugar jarred marinara sauce, divided

Post-Op Servings

Ⓖ 2 rollatinis

1 Preheat the oven to 400°F. Spray 1 or 2 baking sheets with the cooking spray.

2 Slice the eggplant lengthwise into ¼-inch pieces. Lay the slices on a paper towel and sprinkle them with salt. Let them sit for 10 minutes to help release some of the water in the eggplant. Pat dry afterward. It's okay to wipe off some of the salt before baking.

3 Place the eggplant on the baking sheet and bake for 10 minutes. Remove from the oven and set aside to cool. Leave the oven on.

4 Put a large pot over medium-high heat. Heat the olive oil for 1 minute. Add the spinach leaves and cook, stirring occasionally, for about 3 minutes or until wilted. Set aside to let cool.

5 Combine the ricotta, ¼ cup of mozzarella, Parmigiano-Reggiano, egg, and garlic in a medium bowl. Mix well. When the spinach is cool, gently stir it into the cheese mixture.

6 Spread ¼ cup of the marinara sauce across the bottom of an 8-by-8-inch baking dish.

7 Spread the cheese mixture (about 2 tablespoons each) onto each eggplant slice, roll the slice, and place seam-side down in the baking dish. Continue until all eggplant slices are made into roll-ups and placed in the pan.

8 Top the rolled eggplant with the remaining ¼ cup of marinara and ½ cup of mozzarella.

9 Reduce the oven temperature to 350°F. Cover the baking sheets with aluminum foil and bake for 30 minutes. Remove the foil and bake for an additional 10 minutes, or until the cheese is brown and bubbly.

Serving tip: *Pack in even more vegetables by serving over a bed of zucchini noodles or "zoodles."*

Per Serving (2 rollatini): Calories: 160; Total fat: 7g; Protein: 11g; Carbs: 16g; Fiber: 6g; Sugar: 8g; Sodium: 330mg

Curried Eggplant and Chickpea Quinoa

MAKES 8 SERVINGS / PREP TIME: 15 MINUTES / COOK TIME: 20 MINUTES
TOTAL TIME: 35 MINUTES

Seasoning vegetables and vegetarian sources of protein makes them much more delicious. For people who aren't veggie lovers, it can be a complete game-changer. This curried vegetarian recipe is full of antioxidant-loaded spices and nutrient-packed vegetables. Don't be overwhelmed by the long ingredient list. It's super easy to toss together, and the leftovers freeze and reheat well.

4 teaspoons minced garlic

1 teaspoon extra-virgin olive oil

1 large onion, chopped

1 red bell pepper, chopped

1 tablespoon ground cumin

1 teaspoon ground turmeric

2 teaspoons smoked paprika

¼ teaspoon cayenne pepper

½ cup water

1 medium eggplant, cut into ½-inch chunks

1 yellow summer squash, cut into ½-inch chunks

3 tomatoes, diced

1 Place a large skillet over medium-high heat. Sauté the garlic in the olive oil for 1 minute. Add the onion and bell pepper and sauté for 2 to 3 minutes, or until tender.

2 Stir in the cumin, turmeric, paprika, and cayenne pepper and cook for 1 to 2 minutes.

3 Add the water, eggplant, squash, tomatoes, and chickpeas. Cover, reduce the heat to medium-low, and cook for 15 minutes.

4 While the vegetables and chickpeas cook, place the quinoa and broth in a small saucepan over medium-high heat. Cover and bring to a boil. Reduce the heat to low and cook for about 15 minutes, or until all liquid has absorbed. Remove the pan from the heat and fluff the quinoa with a fork. (Otherwise, make the quinoa according to the package instructions.)

1 (15-ounce) can
chickpeas, drained
and rinsed

½ cup packaged quinoa

1 cup vegetable or
chicken broth

Low-fat plain Greek
yogurt, for garnish

Post-Op Servings

Ⓖ 1 cup

5 Serve the curried vegetables over the quinoa, garnished with a dollop of the yogurt.

Post-op tip: *Choose your high-protein grains wisely. Ancient grains like quinoa, millet, barley, and amaranth are loaded with whole-grain protein. Check the label on your whole grains and you might be surprised how packed they can be with nutrient-rich protein.*

Per Serving (1 cup): Calories: 131; Total fat: 2g; Protein: 6g; Carbs: 23g; Fiber: 6g; Sugar: 6g; Sodium: 127mg

Cheesy Cauliflower Casserole

MAKES 8 SERVINGS / PREP TIME: 10 MINUTES / COOK TIME: 45 MINUTES
TOTAL TIME: 55 MINUTES

For the ultimate comfort food, look no farther than mac and cheese. Now that you've joined the VSG Club, traditional mac and cheese, with its high-fat cheese sauce and high-carb pasta, is out of the question. But fear not. This recipe serves up a fantastic meal, sure to please kids and adults of all ages.

1 head cauliflower, cut into florets

1 cup low-fat cottage cheese

1 cup low-fat plain Greek yogurt

½ teaspoon Dijon mustard

¼ teaspoon garlic powder

2 ounces (½ cup) shredded aged white Cheddar cheese

2 ounces (½ cup) shredded mild Cheddar cheese

Post-Op Servings

S ½ cup

G ½ to 1 cup serving

1 Preheat the oven to 350°F.

2 Fill a medium pot one-third full with water, and place a steamer basket inside. Bring the water to a boil over high heat.

3 Add the cauliflower to the steamer basket, cover the pot, and reduce the heat to a gentle boil. Steam the cauliflower for 10 to 15 minutes, or until the florets are soft. Alternatively, you can steam the cauliflower with 2 tablespoons of water in the microwave on high for about 4 minutes, or until tender.

4 While the cauliflower steams, mix together the cottage cheese, yogurt, mustard, and garlic powder in a medium bowl.

5 Drain the cauliflower in a large colander, and gently mash it with a potato masher to drain out excess water.

6 Stir the cauliflower pieces into the cottage cheese mixture. Add the Cheddar cheeses and mix well.

7 Transfer the cauliflower mixture to an 8-by-8-inch or 11-by-7-inch baking dish. Bake for about 30 minutes. It is done when the edges begin to brown.

8 Serve immediately.

Cooking tip: *Instead of your traditional Cheddar cheese, try something with a bit more flavor—Gruyère, smoked Gouda, or Havarti. By using a more flavorful cheese, you may find yourself more satisfied with a smaller portion of the finished recipe.*

Per Serving (½ cup): Calories: 147; Total fat: 7g; Protein: 13g; Carbs: 8g; Fiber: 2g; Sugar: 4g; Sodium: 263g

Butternut Squash and Black Bean Enchiladas

MAKES 8 ENCHILADAS / PREP TIME: 15 MINUTES / COOK TIME: 40 MINUTES
TOTAL TIME: 55 MINUTES

Picture yourself indulging in a cheesy enchilada with all the classic seasonings of typical Mexican food but without the added fat. Does it bring a satisfied smile to your face? These squash and bean enchiladas will satisfy your craving. Try making Homemade Enchilada Sauce (page 175) to pack in even more flavor without all the extra sodium that comes in canned versions. This is a great dish to make ahead and freeze for a dinner after a long day, or for the next time you have dinner guests.

1 teaspoon extra-virgin olive oil

2 teaspoons minced garlic

1 onion, diced

1 jalapeño pepper, seeded and finely diced

1 red bell pepper, finely diced

1 small butternut squash (about 2½ pounds), peeled, seeds removed, and diced

1 teaspoon low-sodium taco seasoning

1 teaspoon ground cumin

1 (10-ounce) can diced tomatoes or 2 large fresh tomatoes, diced

1 (15.5-ounce) can black beans, drained and rinsed

¼ cup water

1 Preheat the oven to 425°F.

2 Place a large skillet (large enough to accommodate all the squash) over medium-high heat. Heat the olive oil and garlic for about 1 minute, or until the garlic is fragrant. Add the onion, jalapeño, and bell pepper. Sauté for 2 to 3 minutes, or until tender.

3 Add the squash, taco seasoning, and cumin. Sauté and stir for 2 minutes, until the seasonings are mixed well. Add the tomatoes, beans, and water. Cover the skillet and cook for 30 minutes, or until squash is tender.

4 Spread ¼ cup of enchilada sauce on the bottom of a 9-by-13-inch baking dish.

5 Place the tortillas on a clean work surface. Fill each tortilla with about ½ cup of the squash mixture. (There may be some left over.) Fold over each tortilla and place them seam-side down in the baking dish.

1 (10-ounce) can red enchilada sauce or about 1 cup Homemade Enchilada Sauce (page 175), divided

8 small whole-wheat tortillas, such as La Tortilla Factory low-carb tortillas

1 cup shredded Monterey Jack cheese

½ cup sliced black olives

2 scallions, chopped

Post-Op Servings

Ⓖ 1 enchilada

6 Pour the remaining (about ¾ cup) enchilada sauce over the top of the enchiladas. Top with the cheese. Cover with aluminum foil.

7 Bake for about 10 minutes, or until cheese is melted.

8 Garnish with the olives and scallions before serving.

Ingredient tip: *Squash is a nutrient-dense vegetable packed with antioxidants like beta-carotene and vitamin C. To save cooking preparation time, purchase squash already peeled and cubed. It can be found in either the fresh or frozen section of your grocery store. Looking for an easy way to bake a fresh butternut squash? Halve the squash, remove and discard the stem, pulp, and seeds, and place the halves cut-side down on a baking sheet coated with the cooking spray. Bake in a preheated 350°F oven for about 45 minutes, or until the flesh is tender and can be mashed or pureed.*

Per Serving (1 enchilada): Calories: 233; Total fat: 8g; Protein: 13g; Carbs: 27g; Fiber: 6g; Sugar: 4g; Sodium: 694mg

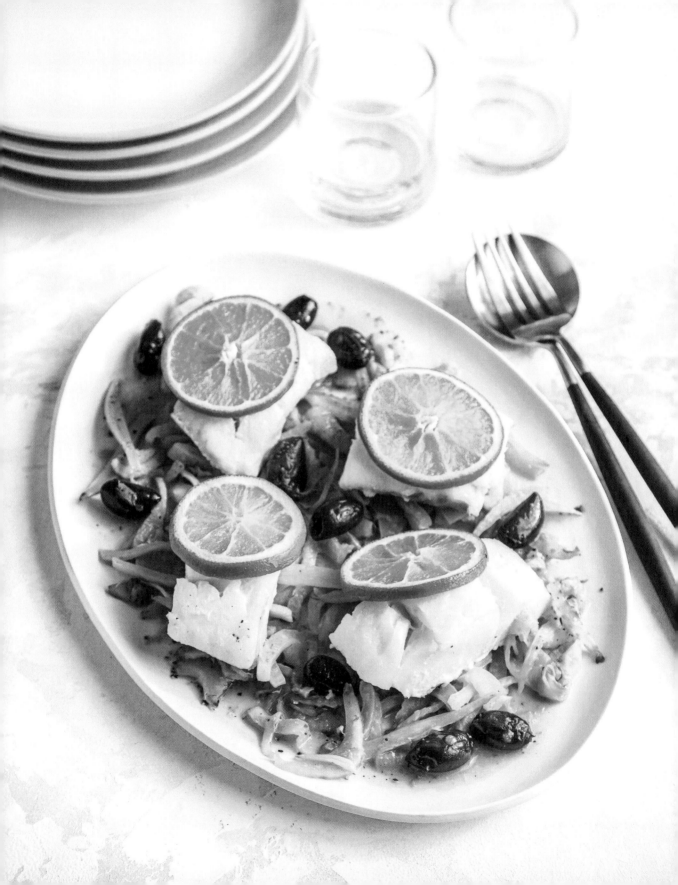

CHAPTER SEVEN

Fish and Seafood Dinners

Tuna Noodle-less Casserole

SERVES 10 / PREP TIME: 15 MINUTES / COOK TIME: 40 MINUTES
TOTAL TIME: 55 MINUTES

Tuna noodle casserole is a classic that's quick to prepare for a weeknight meal. This noodle-less version comes to you via Matt and Diana Luttmann, who are parents of three small children. They always keep the ingredients on hand in their cupboard for a last-minute meal on those extra-busy days. This recipe is so creamy, flavorful, and delicious you won't even know the noodles are missing. The red bell pepper, tomatoes, and green beans give it just a bit of color to make it more interesting than the boring typical beige version.

Nonstick cooking spray

1 medium red onion, chopped

1 red bell pepper, chopped

1½ cups diced tomato

3 cups fresh green beans

⅓ cup olive oil-based mayonnaise

1 (14.5-ounce) can condensed cream of mushroom soup

½ cup low-fat milk

1 cup shredded Cheddar cheese

½ teaspoon freshly ground black pepper

8 (5-ounce) cans water-packed albacore tuna, drained

Post-Op Servings

S ½ cup

G 1 cup

1 Preheat the oven to 425°F.

2 Coat a large skillet with the cooking spray and place it over medium heat. Add the onion, red bell pepper, and tomatoes and sauté for about 5 minutes, or until the vegetables are tender and the tomatoes start to soften. Remove the skillet from the heat and set aside.

3 Cut off the stem ends of the green beans, and snap them into 3- to 4-inch pieces.

4 Fill a large saucepot ⅓ full with water, and place a steamer basket inside. Place the pot over high heat, and bring the water to a boil.

5 Add the green beans to the steamer basket, cover the pot, and reduce the heat to medium. Steam the green beans for 5 minutes. Immediately remove them from the heat, drain, and set aside.

6 Coat a 9-by-13-inch baking dish with the cooking spray.

7 In a large bowl, mix together the mayonnaise, condensed soup, milk, and cheese. Season the mixture with the black pepper.

8 Add the tuna, green beans, and sautéed vegetables to the bowl, and mix to combine. Pour the mixture into the baking dish.

9 Bake for 30 minutes, or until edges start to brown. Serve.

Cooking tip: *It's easy to shake up this standby recipe. To boost protein and reduce fat, add ½ cup of nonfat cottage cheese and reduce the mayonnaise to 2 tablespoons. Use an immersion blender to puree until smooth. To change the flavor profile, first sauté the diced tomatoes in 1 teaspoon of extra-virgin olive oil for 5 minutes before cooking the rest of the vegetables. Set the sautéed tomatoes aside and mix them in with the tuna. Then follow the rest of directions to put together the casserole. The tomatoes become almost like sun-dried and help attenuate some of the fishiness of the tuna.*

Per Serving (1 cup): Calories: 147; Total fat: 7g; Protein: 15g; Carbs: 6g; Fiber: 2g; Sugar: 2g; Sodium: 318mg

Herb-Crusted Salmon

SERVES 2 / PREP TIME: 10 MINUTES / COOK TIME: 20 MINUTES
TOTAL TIME: 30 MINUTES

When it comes to power-packed protein foods, salmon is at the very top of the list. It is one of the best dietary sources of omega-3 fatty acids. Among many benefits, omega-3 fats are important for raising heart-healthy HDL cholesterol and fighting inflammation in the body. This baked salmon recipe will melt in your mouth and even non lovers of fish will delight in its tasty goodness.

2 (4-ounce) salmon fillets
2 teaspoons minced garlic
1 tablespoon dried parsley
½ teaspoon dried thyme
2 teaspoons freshly
   squeezed lemon
4 tablespoons grated
   Parmigiano-
   Reggiano cheese

Post-Op Servings

(S) 2 ounces

(G) 4 ounces

1 Preheat the oven to 425°F. Line a rimmed baking sheet with parchment paper.

2 Place the salmon skin-side down on the baking sheet and cover with a second piece of parchment paper. Bake for 10 minutes.

3 Meanwhile, mix together the garlic, parsley, thyme, lemon juice, and Parmigiano-Reggiano cheese in a small dish.

4 Discard the parchment paper covering the salmon. Use a pastry brush to carefully cover the fillets with the herb-cheese mixture.

5 Bake the salmon, uncovered, for about 5 minutes more. The salmon is done when the fish flakes easily with a fork.

6 Serve immediately.

Cooking tip: *Don't overcook the salmon. Overcooked fish turns rubbery and the "fishy" flavor tends to be empha-sized. Fish is safely cooked when the internal temperature measures 145°F with a meat thermometer.*

Per Serving (4 ounces): Calories: 197; Total fat: 10g; Protein: 27g; Carbs: 9g; Fiber: 1g; Sugar: 3g; Sodium: 222mg

Slow-Roasted Pesto Salmon

SERVES 4 / PREP TIME: 5 MINUTES / COOK TIME: 20 MINUTES
TOTAL TIME: 25 MINUTES

Most people in other countries consume more seafood and fish than most Americans, and not surprisingly also have lower incidence of being overweight and obese. Fish and seafood contain the same amount of protein per ounce as red meat; they're just lower in calories and saturated fat. A fellow dietitian, Michelle McDonagh, who happens to be from the beautiful country of Ireland, brought me this great salmon recipe. It's cooked slowly to help meld the flavors and keep the fish from drying out.

4 (6-ounce) salmon fillets

1 teaspoon extra-virgin olive oil

4 tablespoons Perfect Basil Pesto (page 177)

Post-Op Servings

(S) 2 ounces

(G) 3 to 6 ounces

1 Preheat the oven to 275°F. Line a rimmed baking sheet with aluminum foil and brush the foil with the olive oil.

2 Place the salmon fillets skin-side down on the baking sheet.

3 Spread 1 tablespoon of pesto on each fillet.

4 Roast the salmon for about 20 minutes, or just until opaque in the center.

5 Serve immediately.

Cooking tip: *Enjoy a gourmet meal any night of the week by keeping a bag of freshly frozen wild Alaskan salmon fillets on hand. Look for the kind that are perfectly portioned into individual fillets for easy meal prep—just thaw in the fridge a day or two before needed.*

Per Serving (3 ounces): Calories: 182; Total fat: 10g; Protein: 20g; Carbs: 1g; Fiber: 0g; Sugar: 0g; Sodium: 90mg

Baked Halibut with Tomatoes and White Wine

SERVES 6 / PREP TIME: 5 MINUTES / COOK TIME: 35 MINUTES
TOTAL TIME: 40 MINUTES

After the sleeve gastrectomy, many patients struggle to eat red meat as it is very dense. This halibut recipe is a great alternative to steak. While not nearly as dense as meat, it's still quite hearty. The sweetness of the Vidalia onion balanced with the tart white wine makes this dish extra delicious.

3 tablespoons of
  extra-virgin olive oil
1 Vidalia onion, chopped
1 tablespoon
  minced garlic
1 (10-ounce) container
  grape tomatoes
¾ cup dry white
  wine, divided
3 tablespoons capers
1½ pounds thick-cut
  halibut fillet, deboned
½ teaspoon
  dried oregano
Salt
Freshly ground
  black pepper

Post-Op Servings

 S 2 to 4 ounces

G 4 ounces

1 Preheat the oven to 350°F.

2 In a Dutch oven or large oven-safe skillet over medium-high heat, heat the olive oil. Add the onion and sauté until browned and softened, 3 to 5 minutes.

3 Add the garlic and cook until fragrant, 1 to 2 minutes.

4 Add the tomatoes and cook for 5 minutes, or until they start to soften. Once the tomatoes start to soften, carefully use a potato masher to gently crush the tomatoes just enough to release their juices.

5 Add ½ cup of the wine to the pan and stir. Cook 2 to 3 minutes until slightly thickened. Stir in the capers.

6 Push the vegetables to the sides of the pan leaving the center of the pan open for the fish. Place the fish in the pan and sprinkle it with the oregano, salt, and pepper, then scoop the tomato mixture over the fish.

7 Pour in the remaining ¼ cup of wine.

8 Place in the oven and bake for about 20 minutes, uncovered, or until the fish flakes easily with a fork or reaches an internal temperature of 145°F. Serve.

Per Serving (4 ounces): Calories: 237; Total fat: 10g; Protein: 24g; Carbs: 6g; Fiber: 1g; Sugar: 2g; Sodium: 166mg

Fried-less Friday Fish Fry with Cod

SERVES 4 / PREP TIME: 15 MINUTES / COOK TIME: 10 MINUTES
TOTAL TIME: 25 MINUTES

Where I'm from in Wisconsin, Friday night you will see most people headed out for a fish fry. These dinners can be more than 1,000 calories and are full of saturated fat. Try this version of to save yourself fat and calories without sacrificing taste. A bit of cayenne pepper adds a little spice. For the lemon pepper seasoning, I like Mrs. Dash.

¾ cup corn meal

¾ cup whole-wheat bread crumbs

1½ teaspoons lemon pepper seasoning

½ teaspoon onion powder

½ teaspoon garlic powder

¼ teaspoon ground cayenne pepper

2 eggs

4 (4-ounce) cod fillets

1½ tablespoons extra-virgin olive oil

Post-Op Servings

ⓟ ¼ cup or 2 ounces pureed (try pureeing with Greek yogurt-based tartar sauce for flavor and consistency)

4 ounces

1 Preheat oven to 450°F.

2 Combine cornmeal, bread crumbs, lemon pepper seasoning, onion powder, garlic powder, and cayenne pepper in a large resealable bag. Shake to mix and set aside.

3 In a small bowl, lightly beat the eggs.

4 Carefully add a fish fillet to the bag to coat it with the dry mixture. Next, dip it into the egg, then coat it a second time in the dry mixture. Set aside on a plate and repeat with the remaining fillets.

5 Place a large oven-safe skillet over medium heat. Add the oil and allow it to heat for 1 minute.

6 Carefully add the fish to the skillet. Brown it on one side for 2 minutes and then gently turn to brown the other side for another 2 minutes.

7 Transfer the skillet to the oven. Bake for 6 to 7 minutes, or until golden brown and flaky.

Serving tip: *For a tartar sauce replacement without the added fat, mix together 2 tablespoons low-fat plain Greek yogurt, 1 teaspoon pickle relish, and ½ teaspoon hot sauce.*

Per Serving (4-ounce fillet): Calories: 297; Total fat: 9g; Protein: 27g; Carbs: 28g; Fiber: 3g; Sugar: 0g; Sodium: 576mg

Baked Cod with Fennel and Kalamata Olives

SERVES 4 / PREP TIME: 10 MINUTES / COOK TIME: 35 MINUTES
TOTAL TIME: 45 MINUTES

Fennel is a vegetable commonly used in both Mediterranean and Greek cuisines that has a licorice-like flavor. Fennel is rich in the cancer-protectant antioxidant minerals magnesium and selenium, which can be in short supply after surgery.

2 teaspoons extra-virgin olive oil

1 fennel bulb, sliced paper thin

¼ cup dry white wine

⅛ cup freshly squeezed orange juice

1 teaspoon freshly ground black pepper

4 (4-ounce) cod fillets

4 slices fresh orange (with rind)

¼ cup Kalamata olives, pitted

2 bay leaves

Post-Op Servings

Ⓢ 2 to 4 ounces

Ⓖ 4 ounces

1 Preheat the oven to 400°F.

2 Place a large Dutch oven or oven-safe skillet over medium heat and add the olive oil. Add the fennel and cook, stirring occasionally, until softened, 8 to 10 minutes.

3 Add the wine. Bring it to a simmer and cook for 1 to 2 minutes. Stir in the orange juice and pepper and simmer for 2 minutes more.

4 Remove the skillet from the heat and arrange the cod on top of the fennel mixture. Place the orange slices over the fillets. Position the olives and bay leaves around fish.

5 Roast for 20 minutes, or until fish is opaque. The fish is done when it flakes easily with a fork or reaches an internal temperature of 145°F. Remove the bay leaves prior to serving.

Did You Know? *Olives are a great source of heart-healthy fat. Although portion control is key because they can be calorie dense, olives can bring a pop of flavor to many recipes. Try black olives on a taco salad, Kalamata olives on a Greek-themed pizza or wrap, or place a dish of mixed olives on your charcuterie board for your next dinner party.*

Per Serving (4 ounces): Calories: 186; Total fat: 5g; Protein: 21g; Carbs: 8g; Fiber: 3g; Sugar: 4g; Sodium: 271mg

Red Snapper Veracruz

SERVES 6 / PREP TIME: 20 MINUTES / COOK TIME: 10 MINUTES
TOTAL TIME: 30 MINUTES

Red snapper is a fish native to the Atlantic Ocean and Gulf of Mexico. I love it with this recipe, but you can easily use halibut or cod instead. This is a recipe brought to you by Kathryn Herricks, a friend of mine whose family spends a lot of time cooking fresh fish in Florida. I love their tip to get the best-tasting fish and seafood: "Ask your fishmonger for freshest catch of the day to make a dinner nothing short of delicious!"

10 to 12 multicolored mini bell peppers, stemmed, seeded, and thinly sliced

1 (10-ounce) container cherry tomatoes, halved

1 cup fresh cilantro, roughly chopped

2 tablespoons capers

Juice of 2 limes

2 tablespoons of extra-virgin olive oil

1 jalapeño pepper, stem and seeds removed, finely diced

4 (4-ounce) snapper fillets

Post-Op Servings

Ⓢ 2 to 4 ounces

Ⓖ 4 ounces

1 Preheat a grill to medium-low. Alternatively, preheat the oven to 425°F.

2 In a small mixing bowl, combine the mini bell peppers, tomatoes, cilantro, capers, lime juice, olive oil, and jalapeño pepper to make the salsa. Set aside.

3 Put four large sheets of aluminum foil (about 8½-by-11 inches in size) on a work surface. Place a fish fillet on a foil sheet and top it with one-fourth of the salsa. Fold over the foil so it covers the fish completely, and roll the edges to tightly seal and prevent any air (and liquid) from escaping. Repeat for the remaining three fillets and salsa.

4 Put the foil packets on the grill and close the lid. (The grill temperature should reach no hotter than 450°F.) Cook for 8 to 10 minutes, or until the fish is opaque. The fish is done when it flakes easily with a fork or reaches an internal temperature of 145°F. If using the oven, place the foil packets on a nonstick baking sheet and bake 12 to 15 minutes, or until the fish flakes easily with a fork.

Per Serving (4 ounces): Calories: 161; Total fat: 8g; Protein: 15g; Carbs: 7g; Fiber: 1g; Sugar: 4g; Sodium: 137mg

Lemon-Parsley Crab Cakes

SERVES 4 / PREP TIME: 15 MINUTES, PLUS 30 MINUTES TO CHILL /
COOK TIME: 10 MINUTES TOTAL TIME: 55 MINUTES

Eating seafood doesn't have to be a luxury with these super-easy crab cakes made with canned lump crabmeat available at any grocery store. You can even meal prep ahead of time and whip up these cakes the day before baking to save time. Serve this with the Tomato, Basil, and Cucumber Salad (page 82) on the side.

3 tablespoons whole-wheat bread crumbs

1 egg, lightly beaten

½ teaspoon Dijon mustard

1½ tablespoons olive oil-based mayonnaise

¼ teaspoon ground cayenne pepper

2 teaspoons chopped fresh parsley

Juice of ½ lemon

2 (6-ounce) cans lump crabmeat, drained and cartilage removed

Nonstick cooking spray

Post-Op Servings

S ½ crab cake

G 1 crab cake

1 In a medium bowl, mix together the bread crumbs, egg, mustard, mayonnaise, cayenne pepper, parsley, and lemon juice.

2 Very gently fold in the lump crabmeat.

3 Using a ¼-cup measuring cup, shape the mixture into 4 individual patties. Put the patties in the refrigerator and let sit for 30 minutes.

4 Preheat the oven to 500°F while the crab cakes rest in the refrigerator. Coat a baking sheet with the cooking spray.

5 Place the crab cakes on the baking sheet and bake on the center rack of the oven 10 minutes, or until starting to brown.

6 Serve immediately.

Cooking tip: *Not all crab cakes are created equal. Most restaurant crab cakes are loaded with more bread-crumb filling than crab and are deep-fried in oil. Go for baked, grilled, or broiled fish or seafood when dining out for a guaranteed healthier option.*

Per Serving (1 crab cake): Calories: 148; Total fat: 4g; Protein: 21g; Carbs: 5g; Fiber: 0g; Sugar: 1g; Sodium: 464mg

Shrimp Cocktail Salad

MAKES 4 SERVINGS / PREP TIME: 10 MINUTES / COOK TIME: 5 MINUTES
TOTAL TIME: 15 MINUTES

The post-op diet is an opportunity to venture into trying more baked, boiled, and grilled seafood. Shrimp, scallops, crab, and lobster are all virtually fat free yet loaded with protein. When you see shrimp cocktail on the menu at a restaurant, at the buffet, or as an appetizer at a party—you know it's a safe bet. Here's a recipe for making boiled shrimp at home more flavorful. You can certainly eat them solo with Seafood Sauce (page 174), or try this version tossed on top of a salad with a creamy dressing.

1 lemon, halved and seeded

1 tablespoon black peppercorns

1 teaspoon dried thyme

1 bay leaf

1 pound unpeeled shrimp (31–35 count)

⅓ cup Seafood Sauce (page 174)

3 tablespoons low-fat plain Greek yogurt

¼ cup olive oil-based mayonnaise

1 large head romaine lettuce, chopped

½ seedless cucumber, chopped

Post-Op Servings

P 4 shrimp pureed with 1 tablespoon Seafood Sauce (no lettuce or mayo-based dressing)

G 8 shrimp with ¼ head of lettuce and 3 tablespoons dressing

1 Fill a large pot with water. Squeeze the juice from the lemon halves into the water, and add the black peppercorns, thyme, and bay leaf. Place the pot over high heat and bring to a boil.

2 While the water is heating, create an ice bath by filling a large bowl with ice and water. Set aside.

3 Add the shrimp to the boiling water and cook them for 2 to 3 minutes, or until they just turn pink.

4 Drain the shrimp in a colander and immediately put them in the ice bath to cool.

5 Once cool, peel the shrimp and remove the tails.

6 In a large bowl, combine the seafood sauce, yogurt, and mayonnaise. Mix well.

7 Add the cooked shrimp to the dressing and stir to coat.

8 Divide the lettuce among 4 plates. Add the cucumber and top it with the dressed shrimp.

9 Serve immediately.

Per Serving (8 shrimp with ¼ head of lettuce and 3 tablespoons dressing): Calories: 163; Total fat: 6g; Protein: 17g; Carbs: 4g; Fiber: 1g; Sugar: 4g; Sodium: 650mg

Seafood Cioppino

SERVES 8 / PREP TIME: 15 MINUTES / COOK TIME: 45 MINUTES
TOTAL TIME: 60 MINUTES

Seafood cioppino is a light meal even without a bariatric-friendly makeover. It's packed with flavorful herbs, high-protein seafood, and a light tomato broth. If you are in the great city of San Francisco and you see this on the menu at a restaurant, you can safely order it and you won't be disappointed! Here is a recipe for making cioppino at home. My best tip: The longer it simmers, the more the flavors meld, so make sure you allow enough time before your dinner will be served.

2 teaspoons minced garlic

1 tablespoon extra-virgin olive oil

2 leeks, washed and cut into ⅛-inch slices, both white and green parts

2 celery stalks, cut into ¼-inch pieces

1 green bell pepper, diced

4 cups water

1½ cups dry white wine

1 (10-ounce) container grape tomatoes

1 large tomato, chopped into ¼-inch pieces

½ teaspoon dried thyme

½ teaspoon dried basil

1 bay leaf

1 tablespoon chopped fresh parsley

Juice of ½ lemon

2 pounds shrimp, deveined

1 (6-ounce) can lump crabmeat, drained and cartilage removed

½ pound scallops

1 teaspoon freshly ground black pepper

1 Place a large pot or Dutch oven over medium heat. Sauté the garlic in the olive oil for 1 to 2 minutes. Add the leeks and stir for about 2 minutes, or until tender.

2 Add the celery and green pepper and cook for about 5 minutes, or until tender.

3 Pour in the water, wine, tomatoes, thyme, basil, bay leaf, parsley, and lemon juice. Bring to a boil, then cover, reduce the heat to low, and let simmer for 25 minutes.

Post-Op Servings

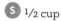 ½ cup

G 1 cup

4 Remove and discard the bay leaf. Add the shrimp, crabmeat, and scallops. Bring back to a simmer and cook for 5 to 10 minutes, or until the shrimp are no longer pink and the scallops are opaque. Stir in the black pepper.

5 Ladle into soup bowls and serve.

Cooking tip: *Add a pound of fresh mussels or even some white fish to include even more variety in this seafood stew. Serve with homemade croutons made from whole-wheat bread if you can tolerate them.*

Per Serving (1 cup): Calories: 171; Total fat: 4g; Protein: 21g; Carbs: 5g; Fiber: 0g; Sugar: 1g; Sodium: 464mg

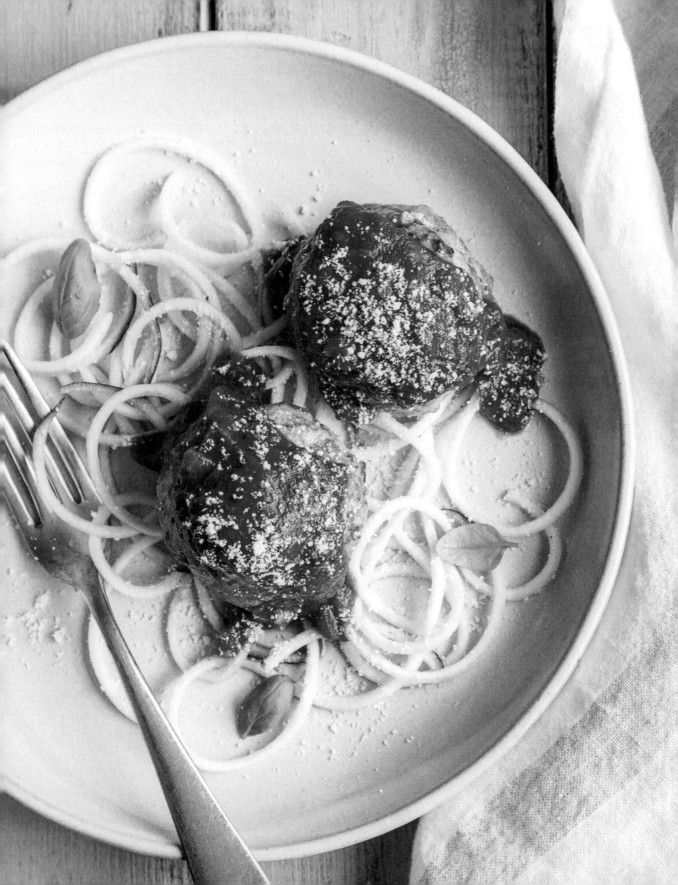

CHAPTER EIGHT

Poultry Dinners

Baked Potato Soup

MAKES 6 SERVINGS / PREP TIME: 10 MINUTES / COOK TIME: 30 MINUTES
TOTAL TIME: 40 MINUTES

Potatoes often get a bad rap for being high in carbohydrates and high in calories, but on the flip side, they are loaded with potassium and rich in fiber, among other nutrients. It's not so much the potato, but what we put on the potato that can make them less than favorable for the waistline. Soups are a fantastic way to fill up on fewer calories because the majority is liquid. Try this creamy baked potato soup. It can feed your family, or you can freeze leftovers in individual containers and use for lunches all week long.

4 slices turkey bacon
(nitrate-free)

2 tablespoons extra-virgin
olive oil

3 tablespoons
whole-wheat flour

1½ cups 1% milk

1½ cups vegetable or
chicken broth

3 medium unpeeled
russet potatoes, cut into
1-inch chunks

½ cup low-fat plain
Greek yogurt

½ cup shredded sharp
Cheddar cheese

4 tablespoons
chopped chives

Post-Op Servings

P ¼ cup

S ½ cup

G 1 to 2 cups

1 Place a large stock pot over medium heat. Add the bacon and cook until crispy on both sides, turning once, about 5 minutes total. Transfer to a paper towel-lined plate to absorb any excess grease. Once cooled, chop finely and set aside.

2 Heat the olive oil in the stock pot over medium heat. Add the flour and cook, stirring constantly, until browned, 2 to 3 minutes. Add the milk and whisk constantly until it starts to thicken. Whisk in the broth.

3 Add the potatoes. Bring to a boil, then reduce the heat to low and let the soup simmer for about 20 minutes, or until the potatoes are tender.

4 Add the Greek yogurt and stir to combine.

5 Serve garnished with the turkey bacon, cheese, chives, and additional dollop of plain Greek yogurt.

Post-op tip: *If you are cooking this during the post-op pureed stage, add 1 to 2 tablespoons of egg white powder or unflavored protein powder after cooking to increase the protein content.*

Per Serving (1 cup): Calories: 181; Total fat: 9g; Protein: 9g; Carbs: 18g; Fiber: 3g; Sugar: 1g; Sodium: 174mg

Creamy Chicken Soup with Cauliflower

MAKES 8 CUPS / PREP TIME: 15 MINUTES / COOK TIME: 40 MINUTES
TOTAL TIME: 55 MINUTES

Giving up restaurant dining and cooking more healthy meals at home doesn't mean giving up on taste and flavor. Quite the opposite. Try this knock-off version of Olive Garden's Chicken & Gnocchi Soup; it has less fat, less sodium, and fewer carbohydrates. Use leftover cooked chicken to save on meal prep time. Grill or bake several servings of chicken breast on the weekend to use for meals throughout the week. You can even substitute canned chicken breast to save on time.

1 teaspoon minced garlic

1 teaspoon extra-virgin olive oil

½ yellow onion, diced

1 carrot, diced

1 celery stalk, diced

1½ pounds (3 or 4 medium) cooked chicken breast, diced

2 cups low-sodium chicken broth

2 cups water

1 teaspoon freshly ground black pepper

1 teaspoon dried thyme

2½ cups fresh cauliflower florets

1 cup fresh spinach, chopped

2 cups nonfat or 1% milk

Post-Op Servings

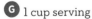 1 cup serving

1 Place a large soup pot over medium-high heat. Sauté the garlic in the olive oil for 1 minute.

2 Add the onion, carrot, and celery and sauté until tender, 3 to 5 minutes.

3 Add the chicken breast, broth, water, black pepper, thyme, and cauliflower. Bring to a simmer, reduce the heat to medium-low, and cook, uncovered, for 30 minutes.

4 Add the fresh spinach and stir until wilted, about 5 minutes.

5 Stir in the milk, then serve immediately.

Did You Know? *Greens such as spinach, kale, and Swiss chard are all excellent sources of iron. Iron is a key nutrient for the red blood cell function of carrying oxygen to cells throughout the body. Add greens at the end of cooking soups and stews as they wilt quickly. It's a great way to use up salad greens that might be on the edge of going bad in your fridge.*

Per Serving (1 cup): Calories: 164; Total fat: 3g; Protein: 25g; Carbs: 5g; Fiber: 1g; Sugar: 4g; Sodium: 54mg

Chicken, Barley, and Vegetable Soup

MAKES 8 CUPS / PREP TIME: 15 MINUTES / COOK TIME: 50 MINUTES
TOTAL TIME: 65 MINUTES

Think classic chicken noodle soup with a twist. Barley instead of noodles gives this soup a bit more texture and makes it more filling. The cooked vegetables are tender and easy on the stomach yet still packed with nutritious anti-oxidants, vitamins, and minerals. Best part: It's even better the next day as the flavors have time to meld. You can freeze this soup in small containers to eat for lunch whenever you need a quick, warm, and filling meal.

1 tablespoon extra-virgin olive oil

1 teaspoon minced garlic

1 large onion, diced

2 large carrots, chopped

3 celery stalks, chopped

1 (14.5-ounce) can diced tomatoes

¾ cup pearl barley

2½ cups diced cooked chicken, such as leftovers from Whole Herbed Roasted Chicken in the Slow Cooker (page 136)

4 cups low-sodium chicken broth

2 cups water

½ teaspoon dried thyme

½ teaspoon dried sage

¼ teaspoon dried rosemary

2 bay leaves

1 Place a large soup pot over medium-high heat. Sauté the olive oil and garlic for 1 minute.

2 Add the onion, carrots, and celery and sauté until tender, 3 to 5 minutes.

3 Add the tomatoes, barley, chicken, broth, water, thyme, sage, rosemary, and bay leaves. Bring to a simmer, then reduce the heat to medium-low and cook, uncovered, for about 45 minutes. The soup is done when the barley is tender.

4 Remove and discard bay leaves before serving.

Per Serving (1 cup): Calories: 198; Total fat: 3g; Protein: 16g; Carbs: 9g; Fiber: 2g; Sugar: 3g; Sodium: 528mg

Post-Op Servings

 1 cup

Slow Cooker Turkey Chili

SERVES 16 / PREP TIME: 10 MINUTES / COOK TIME: 8 HOURS
TOTAL TIME: 8 HOURS, 10 MINUTES

Chili is a simple meal to make, it has loads of flavor, and it seems to go down well post-op. Once the chili is cooked, feel free to garnish it with plain low-fat Greek yogurt, low-fat shredded Cheddar cheese, and chopped scallions. Keep the canned ingredients in your cupboard so you can quickly toss together this meal. This recipe is brought to you by Amy Kulwicki, RD.

Nonstick cooking spray

2 pounds extra-lean
  ground turkey

2 (14.5-ounce) cans kidney
  beans, drained
  and rinsed

1 (28-ounce) can diced
  tomatoes with
  green chiles

1 (8-ounce) can
  tomato puree

1 large onion,
  finely chopped

1 green bell pepper,
  finely chopped

2 celery stalks,
  finely chopped

4 teaspoons minced garlic

1 teaspoon dried oregano

2 tablespoons
  ground cumin

3 tablespoons
  chili powder

1 (8-ounce) can
  tomato juice

1 Place a large skillet over medium-high heat and coat it with the cooking spray. Add the ground turkey. Using a wooden spoon, break it into smaller pieces and cook until browned, 7 to 9 minutes.

2 While the turkey browns, place the beans, tomatoes, tomato puree, onion, bell pepper, celery, garlic, oregano, cumin, chili powder, and tomato juice in the slow cooker. Stir in the cooked ground turkey and mix well.

3 Cover the slow cooker and turn on low to cook for 8 hours.

4 Serve garnished with Greek yogurt, shredded Cheddar cheese, and chopped scallions (if using).

Per Serving (½ cup): Calories: 140; Total fat: 4g; Protein: 14g; Carbs: 12g; Fiber: 4g; Sugar: 4g; Sodium: 280mg

Post-Op Servings

P ¼ cup

S ¼ to ½ cup

G ½ to 1 cup

Slow Cooker White Chicken Chili

SERVES 6 / PREP TIME: 10 MINUTES / COOK TIME: 6 HOURS
TOTAL TIME: 6 HOURS, 10 MINUTES

Hearty soups and chilis fill you up from inside out and they're great ways to pack plenty of vegetables and protein into your post-op diet. Many creamy soups are made with rich cheese or heavy cream. Try this version, which uses pureed beans to give the chili its creamy texture.

2 (14.5-ounce) cans chickpeas, drained and rinsed, divided

2 cups low-sodium chicken broth, divided

1 pound boneless, skinless chicken breasts

1 large onion, diced

1 jalapeño pepper, seeded, minced

1 tablespoon ground cumin

1½ teaspoons ground coriander

2 teaspoons dried oregano

2 teaspoons chili powder

1 (4-ounce) can diced green chiles

2 cups water

¼ cup chopped cilantro, for garnish (optional)

1 Prepare bean puree. In a blender or food processor, blend 1 can of the beans with 1 cup of broth. Set aside.

2 Place the chicken breasts in a 4- or 6-quart slow cooker. Top them with the onion, jalapeño, cumin, coriander, oregano, chili powder, and green chiles.

3 Add the remaining 1 cup of broth, water, remaining 1 can of beans, and bean puree.

4 Cover the slow cooker, turn on low, and set the timer for 6 hours. At the 5½-hour mark, transfer the chicken to a plate and shred it with a fork. Return it to the slow cooker, and continue cooking on low for an additional 20 to 30 minutes before serving, allowing the chicken to absorb some of the liquid.

5 Ladle into bowls to serve and garnish with the cilantro.

Post-Op Servings

P ¼ cup (2 ounces)

S ½ cup (4 ounces)

G 4 ounces

Post-op tip: *Eating spicy foods might help with your weight loss. When eating foods with a little extra-spicy kick, you might find you feel more satiated and eat less. The verdict is still out as to whether spicy peppers can speed your metabolism—but adding a little extra jalapeño to your chili might help you slow down and savor your meal. Bonus: Jalapeños are packed with lots of antioxidants.*

Per Serving (1 cup): Calories: 225; Total fat: 3g; Protein: 26g; Carbs: 25g; Fiber: 7g; Sugar: 3g; Sodium: 661mg

DZ's Grilled Chicken Wings

MAKES ABOUT 18 WINGS / PREP TIME: 15 MINUTES / COOK TIME: 20 MINUTES
TOTAL TIME: 35 MINUTES

Whether it's for a Super Bowl party, Sunday afternoon picnic, or just a week-night dinner—hot wings are always a fan-favorite. Most wings are breaded and deep-fried, then dredged in some sort of sugar-packed barbecue sauce. These juicy wings are grilled to perfection so the chicken falls right off the bone! Choose a buffalo wing sauce with a heat that's appropriate for you. Flaming hot sauce is optional—but go for it if that's your thing! This recipe is brought to you by grillmaster Dan Zangerle, whose famous grilled wings are always a favorite when guests are at his home.

1½ pounds frozen
 chicken wings

Freshly ground
 black pepper

1 teaspoon garlic powder

1 cup buffalo wing sauce,
 such as Frank's RedHot

1 teaspoon extra-virgin
 olive oil

Post-Op Servings

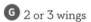 **G** 2 or 3 wings

1 Preheat the grill to 350°F.

2 Season the wings with the black pepper and garlic powder.

3 Grill the wings for 15 minutes per side. They will be browned and crispy when finished.

4 Toss the grilled wings in the buffalo wing sauce and olive oil.

5 Serve immediately.

Post-op tip: *Go for the meat and skip the skin whenever possible. In the early days, weeks, and months post-op, most people will not tolerate the skin on chicken or turkey because of its dense texture. After 6 to 9 months, eating 2 or 3 deep-fried chicken wings with the skin may be tolerated, but limit portions when possible because of the high saturated fat content. Remember, everything in moderation. If wings are your favorite, you are a step ahead with this grilled version.*

Per Serving (1 wing): Calories: 82; Total fat: 6g; Protein: 7g; Carbs: 1g; Fiber: 0g; Sugar: 0g; Sodium: 400mg

Ranch-Seasoned Crispy Chicken Tenders

MAKES 6 CHICKEN TENDERS / PREP TIME: 10 MINUTES / COOK TIME: 20 MINUTES
TOTAL TIME: 30 MINUTES

Be cautious anytime you consider eating something with the word nugget *or* finger *in the title after* chicken. *More than likely you're getting a whole lot of crispy fried coating and not a lot of lean chicken breast. Skip the fast-food versions and make these chicken tenders at home. The crispy coating helps hold in all the juices to keep the chicken moist with every bite. Serve with a side of roasted vegetables or dip them in Creamy Peppercorn Ranch Dressing (page 173).*

Nonstick cooking spray

6 chicken tenderloin pieces (about 1¼ pounds)

2 tablespoons whole-wheat pastry flour

1 egg, lightly beaten

½ cup whole-wheat bread crumbs

2 tablespoons grated Parmigiano-Reggiano cheese

2 teaspoons dried parsley

¾ teaspoon dried dill

¼ teaspoon garlic powder

¼ teaspoon onion powder

¼ teaspoon dried basil

⅛ teaspoon freshly ground black pepper

Post-Op Servings

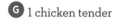 1 chicken tender

1 Preheat the oven to 425°F. Spray a baking sheet with the cooking spray.

2 Prepare three small dishes for coating the chicken. Place the flour in one, the egg in the second, and in the last dish mix together the bread crumbs, Parmigiano-Reggiano cheese, parsley, dill, garlic powder, onion powder, basil, and black pepper.

3 Working one at a time, dip each tenderloin into the flour. Shake off any excess, then dip the chicken into the egg. Finally, place the tenderloin in the bread crumbs and press to coat in the mixture. Place on the baking sheet.

4 Bake for about 20 minutes, or until crispy, brown and cooked through. Serve immediately.

Serving tip: *Turn these into a Buffalo ranch chicken salad. Toss the crispy tenders with Frank's RedHot Buffalo Wing Sauce. Chop and place on top of a salad of mixed greens, shredded carrots, and tomatoes and top with low-fat blue cheese. Drizzle the salad with the Creamy Peppercorn Ranch Dressing (page 173).*

Per Serving (1 chicken tender): Calories: 162; Total fat: 2g; Protein: 25g; Carbs: 8g; Fiber: 1g; Sugar: 1g; Sodium: 239mg

Chicken "Nachos" with Sweet Bell Peppers

MAKES ABOUT 16 "NACHOS" / PREP TIME: 10 MINUTES / COOK TIME: 25 MINUTES / TOTAL TIME: 35 MINUTES

Make a simple swap of fried tortilla chips for crispy, sweet bell peppers. No one will notice the chips are missing!

Nonstick cooking spray

1 (1-pound) package mini bell peppers, stemmed, seeded, and halved

2 teaspoons extra-virgin olive oil

½ onion, minced

2 cups cooked shredded chicken breast (see Ingredient tip)

1 large tomato, diced

1 teaspoon garlic powder

1 teaspoon ground cumin

½ teaspoon smoked paprika

1 cup shredded Colby Jack cheese

¼ cup sliced black olives

3 scallions, finely sliced

1 jalapeño pepper, seeded, thinly sliced (optional)

Post-Op Servings

G 2 mini bell pepper halves

1 Preheat the oven to 400°F. Line a baking sheet with aluminum foil and coat the foil with the cooking spray.

2 Arrange the bell pepper halves on the baking sheet cut-side up.

3 Heat the olive oil in a large skillet over medium heat. Add the onion and sauté for 1 to 2 minutes, or until tender. Add the chicken, tomato, garlic powder, cumin, and paprika and cook for about 5 minutes, or until the tomato has softened and the chicken is heated through.

4 Spoon 1 heaping tablespoon of the chicken mixture into each mini bell pepper half. Top each with the cheese, black olives, scallions, and jalapeño (if using).

5 Bake for 15 minutes, or until cheese has melted and browned. Enjoy immediately.

Ingredient tip: *For the chicken, you can shred leftovers from the Whole Herbed Roasted Chicken in the Slow Cooker (page 136) or buy a rotisserie chicken.*

Serving tip: *Turn these nachos into a well-rounded meal by serving with a side of Refried Black Beans (page 58) and topping with some fresh avocado slices.*

Per Serving (2 mini stuffed bell pepper halves): Calories: 189; Total fat: 3g; Protein: 29g; Carbs: 9g; Fiber: 2g; Sugar: 2g; Sodium: 143mg

Buffalo Chicken Wrap

MAKES 5 WRAPS / PREP TIME: 15 MINUTES / TOTAL TIME: 15 MINUTES

Doughy bread is not always the friend of many post-op patients. Enter the wrap as an excellent alternative. There are many varieties out there that are low in calories and carbohydrates. Some come in at 90 calories or less, which is the equivalent of 1 slice of bread. This Buffalo chicken wrap is made with grilled chicken and is a great choice in place of the typical versions at your local eatery, which are usually loaded with deep-fried chicken. You can always make this a "naked" wrap and do without the outer shell.

3 cups cooked grilled, canned, or rotisserie chicken breast

2 cups chopped romaine lettuce

1 tomato, diced

½ red onion, finely sliced

¼ cup Buffalo wing sauce, such as Frank's RedHot

¼ cup Creamy Peppercorn Ranch Dressing (page 173)

Chopped raw celery (optional)

5 small 100% whole-grain low-carb wraps, such as Tumaro's low-carb wraps

1 In a large mixing bowl, combine the chicken, lettuce, tomato, onion, wing sauce, dressing, and celery (if using).

2 Place about 1 cup of the mixture onto each wrap. Fold the wrap over the top of the salad, close in the sides, and then tightly roll the wrap closed. Use a toothpick to secure the wrap, if needed, and serve.

Per Serving (1 wrap): Calories: 200; Total fat: 7g; Protein: 28g; Carbs: 14g; Fiber: 8g; Sugar: 2g; Sodium: 503 mg

Post-Op Servings

 1 wrap

Jerk Chicken with Mango Salsa

SERVES 4 / PREP TIME: 15 MINUTES, PLUS 30 MINUTES TO MARINADE
COOK TIME: 15 MINUTES / TOTAL TIME: 1 HOUR

Set the burgers and hot dogs aside and try this jerk chicken recipe for your next summer barbecue. The smoky seasonings and refreshing mango salsa will have you and your guests feeling like you are on the beach in Jamaica. You can even put on some calypso music to get everyone in the mood. This is great served over Cauliflower Rice (page 85).

2 tablespoons extra-virgin olive oil

Juice of 1 lime

1 tablespoon minced garlic

1 teaspoon ground ginger

½ teaspoon dried thyme

½ teaspoon cinnamon

½ teaspoon ground allspice

½ teaspoon ground nutmeg

¼ teaspoon cayenne pepper

¼ teaspoon ground cloves

1 teaspoon freshly ground black pepper

4 boneless, skinless chicken breasts about (1 pound chicken)

1 cup Mango Salsa (page 176)

1 In a gallon-size zip-top freezer bag, put the olive oil, lime juice, garlic, ginger, thyme, cinnamon, allspice, nutmeg, cayenne, cloves, and black pepper. Tightly seal the bag and gently mix the marinade.

2 Add the chicken breasts to the marinade. Tightly seal the bag and shake to coat the chicken in the marinade.

3 Refrigerate for at least 30 minutes or overnight.

4 Preheat the grill to medium-high heat. Place the chicken on the grill and discard the marinade. Cook the chicken for about 6 minutes on each side or until the breasts are no longer pink in the middle and reach an internal temperature of 165°F. Alternatively, bake the chicken in a preheated 400°F oven for about 25 minutes, or until the juices run clear.

5 Let the chicken rest for 5 minutes before slicing. Top the chicken slices with the Mango Salsa.

Post-Op Servings

Ⓖ 4 ounces with ¼ cup Mango Salsa

Per Serving (4 ounces): Calories: 206; Total fat: 9g; Protein: 25g; Carbs: 11g; Fiber: 1g; Sugar: 9g; Sodium: 111mg

Baked "Fried Chicken" Thighs

SERVES 4 / PREP TIME: 10 MINUTES / COOK TIME: 35 MINUTES
TOTAL TIME: 45 MINUTES

Fried chicken is the most popular meal to order in a restaurant in the United States, but it's laden with artery-clogging fat and will certainly not be well tolerated by your new stomach after surgery. Try this tasty baked recipe, which is loaded with flavor and has a crunchy coating made from cereal that will make you think it was deep-fried.

Nonstick cooking spray
1 teaspoon
    smoked paprika
½ teaspoon garlic powder
½ teaspoon freshly
    ground black pepper
½ teaspoon
    cayenne pepper
½ teaspoon
    dried oregano
4 (5-ounce) boneless,
    skinless chicken thighs
2 large eggs
1 tablespoon water
1 teaspoon Dijon mustard
2½ cups bran flakes

Post-Op Servings

Ⓢ ½ chicken thigh
(2 to 4 ounces)

Ⓖ 1 chicken thigh
(4 to 6 ounces)

1 Preheat the oven to 400°F. Line a large rimmed baking sheet with aluminum foil, and place it in the oven below a clean oven rack. Spray the clean rack with the cooking spray.

2 In a large zip-top bag, combine the paprika, garlic powder, black pepper, cayenne pepper, and oregano. Add the chicken thighs to the bag, seal the bag, and shake to coat the thighs with the seasonings. Set aside.

3 In a small bowl, lightly whisk together the eggs, water, and mustard.

4 Crush the bran flakes in another large plastic bag.

5 To bread the chicken, dredge the seasoned chicken thighs in the egg mixture, and then put them in the bag of crushed cereal. Shake to coat well.

6 Place the chicken thighs on the clean oven rack, making sure the baking sheet is directly under the chicken to catch any drippings.

7 Bake for 35 minutes, or until the thighs are crispy and reach an internal temperature of 165°F, and serve.

Post-op tip: *Dark meat chicken is slightly higher in saturated fat than its white meat counterpart, but don't fear trying the dark meat, since it tends to be more moist and tender than chicken breast. After surgery, a soft texture is very important to being able to tolerate different proteins. Balance out this meal by serving it with Cheesy Cauliflower Casserole (page 100) and your choice of vegetables.*

Per Serving (1 chicken thigh): Calories: 272; Total fat: 8g; Protein: 35g; Carbs: 15g; Fiber: 3g; Sugar: 3g; Sodium: 279mg

Egg Roll in a Bowl

SERVES 6 / PREP TIME: 10 MINUTES / COOK TIME: 20 MINUTES
TOTAL TIME: 30 MINUTES

Chinese food is no longer a meal of the past with this quick go-to recipe—there's far less fat in it than most takeout meals. Enjoy the flavors of an egg roll without the fried coating. Make this one-pot meal and save the leftovers for lunch or dinner the next day.

2 teaspoons sesame oil, divided

1 teaspoon minced garlic

1 onion, finely diced

1 pound extra-lean ground chicken or turkey

1½ tablespoons low-sodium soy sauce or Bragg Liquid Aminos

½ cup low-sodium beef broth

2 teaspoons ground ginger

½ teaspoon freshly ground black pepper

4 cups green cabbage, chopped or shredded into 1-inch ribbons

1½ cups shredded carrots

1 cup fresh bean sprouts or 1 (14-ounce) can, drained and rinsed

2 scallions, finely chopped, for garnish

1   Place a large skillet over medium-high heat. Add 1 teaspoon of sesame oil and the garlic. Stir for 1 minute. Add the onion and cook until tender, 1 to 2 minutes. Add the ground chicken. Cook until browned, breaking up the meat into smaller pieces, 7 to 9 minutes.

2   While the meat is browning, mix together the remaining 1 teaspoon of the sesame oil, soy sauce, broth, ginger, and black pepper in a small bowl.

3   When the chicken is cooked, stir the sauce into the skillet. Add the cabbage, carrots, and bean sprouts. Stir to combine. Cover the skillet and simmer until the cabbage is tender, 5 to 7 minutes.

4   Serve in a bowl and garnish with the scallions and additional soy sauce to taste.

Prep tip: *Cut preparation time in half by purchasing a prepackaged bag of coleslaw mix to use in place of chopping your own cabbage and carrots.*

Post-Op Servings

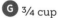 ¾ cup

Per Serving (¾ cup): Calories: 133; Total fat: 3g; Protein: 19g; Carbs: 7g; Fiber 2g; Sugars: 4g; Sodium: 356mg

Chicken Cordon Bleu

MAKES 6 SERVINGS / PREP TIME: 15 MINUTES / COOK TIME: 30 MINUTES / TOTAL
TIME: 45 MINUTES

*By now you've figured out that getting in enough protein is the main theme of
the post-op sleeve diet. Focusing on lean sources of protein such as chicken
and fish are important to keep calories down. Try this healthier twist on a
classic chicken recipe. The light coating helps hold in the moisture when the
chicken bakes. Serve with a side of the Barley-Mushroom Risotto (page 93).*

Nonstick cooking spray

6 boneless, skinless
chicken breasts (about
3 ounces each),
thinly sliced

6 slices lean deli ham
(nitrate-free; about
5 ounces total)

6 slices reduced-fat Swiss
cheese (3 ounces
total), halved

2 large eggs

1 tablespoon water

¼ cup whole-wheat
bread crumbs

2 tablespoons grated
Parmigiano-
Reggiano cheese

Post-Op Servings

Ⓖ 1 chicken breast

1 Preheat the oven to 450°F. Spray a baking sheet
with the cooking spray.

2 Pound the chicken breasts to ¼-inch thickness.

3 Layer 1 slice of ham and 1 slice (2 halves) of cheese
on each chicken breast. Carefully roll the chicken.
Place it seam-side down on the baking sheet.

4 In a small bowl, lightly whisk the eggs. In a second
small bowl, mix together the bread crumbs and
Parmigiano-Reggiano cheese.

5 Using a pastry brush, lightly brush each chicken
roll with the egg wash and then sprinkle on the
bread-crumb mixture.

6 Bake for 30 minutes, or until the chicken is cooked
thoroughly and lightly browned on top.

Per Serving (1 chicken breast): Calories: 174; Total fat: 7g;
Protein: 24g; Carbs: 3g; Fiber: 0g; Sugar: 0g; Sodium: 321mg

Zoodles with Turkey Meatballs

SERVES 4 / PREP TIME: 15 MINUTES / COOK TIME: 20 MINUTES
TOTAL TIME: 35 MINUTES

Cutting down on carbs after surgery means avoiding pasta, but that doesn't mean you have to go without spaghetti and meatballs. You just have to think about spaghetti in a different way. Try this version of "spaghetti" made with zoodles (zucchini noodles). Using ground turkey instead of beef is a simple swap, but when mixed with the flavorful sauce, onion, and bread crumbs, no one will know the difference.

Nonstick cooking spray

1 large egg

½ cup whole-wheat
   bread crumbs

⅓ cup chopped onion

½ teaspoon freshly
   ground black pepper

1 pound extra-lean
   ground turkey

1 pound zucchini (about
   3 medium zucchini)

1 teaspoon extra-virgin
   olive oil

2 cups Marinara Sauce
   with Italian Herbs
   (page 178), or a
   low-sugar jarred
   marinara sauce

Post-Op Servings

S 1 meatball with
2 ounces sauce

G 2 meatballs with 2 to
4 ounces sauce and
¼ cup zoodles

1 Preheat the oven to 400°F. Coat the bottom of a shallow baking pan with the cooking spray.

2 In a large bowl, combine the egg, bread crumbs, onion, and pepper.

3 Add the ground turkey and using clean hands, mix well until the mixture is evenly distributed.

4 Shape the meat mixture into 2-inch balls and place in the baking pan.

5 Bake, uncovered, for 15 minutes.

6 Cut off the ends of the zucchini. Use a mandolin, spiralizer, or the side of a box grater to slice the zucchini into long, thin strips.

7 In a medium skillet over medium heat, heat the olive oil. Add the zucchini strips and sauté for about 5 minutes, or until tender. Transfer to a serving bowl.

8 Serve the meatballs over the zoodles and top with the marinara sauce.

Per Serving (2 meatballs with 2 ounces sauce and ¼ cup zoodles):
Calories: 191; Total fat: 5g; Protein: 22g; Carbs: 15g; Fiber: 3g; Sugar: 4g; Sodium: 205mg

Slow Cooker Barbecue Shredded Chicken

SERVES 4 / PREP TIME: 5 MINUTES / COOK TIME: 6½ TO 8½ HOURS
TOTAL TIME: 6½ TO 8½ HOURS

This melt-in-your-mouth savory chicken dish is delicious in a wrap or on top of a baked potato—and all on its own, of course. Batch cook several chicken breasts to make enough meat to freeze for later use, serve a crowd, or use throughout the week with different meal options.

4 (4-ounce) boneless, skinless chicken breasts

1 cup catsup (free of high-fructose corn syrup)

½ cup water

1 tablespoon freshly squeezed lemon juice

1 tablespoon dried onions

½ teaspoon dried mustard

¼ teaspoon red pepper flakes

3 tablespoons Worcestershire sauce

1 tablespoon white vinegar

Post-Op Servings

Ⓟ ¼ cup (2 ounces)

Ⓢ ½ cup (4 ounces)

Ⓖ ½ cup (4 ounces)

1 Place the chicken breasts in a slow cooker.

2 In a small bowl, whisk together the catsup, water, lemon juice, dried onions, dried mustard, red pepper flakes, Worcestershire sauce, and white vinegar. Pour the mixture over the chicken.

3 Cover the slow cooker and turn on low to cook for 6 to 8 hours.

4 Transfer the chicken to a plate and shred it with a fork. Return it to the slow cooker, and cook on low for 30 minutes more before serving, allowing the chicken to absorb some of the liquid.

Per Serving (4 ounces): Calories: 188; Total fat: 3g; Protein: 22g; Carbs: 16g; Fiber: 0g; Sugar: 10g; Sodium: 750mg

Whole Herbed Roasted Chicken in the Slow Cooker

SERVES 6 / PREP TIME: 15 MINUTES / COOK TIME: 7 HOURS
TOTAL TIME: 7 HOURS, 15 MINUTES

Toss a whole chicken in the slow cooker for a quick easy meal that's done when you get home from work. Everyone in the family is happy because you have plenty of both white and dark meat to please all chicken lovers. The best part about cooking this whole chicken is that leftovers can easily be made into soups, casseroles, or stir fries. Whether you are cooking for one or for an entire family, cooking a whole chicken is a win-win.

1 teaspoon garlic powder

1 teaspoon smoked paprika

1 teaspoon onion powder

1 teaspoon dried thyme

½ teaspoon freshly ground black pepper

½ teaspoon dried sage

1 (4-pound) whole chicken

2 sprigs fresh rosemary

2 lemon wedges

Post-Op Servings

Ⓟ ¼ cup (2 ounces)

Ⓢ ½ cup (4 ounces)

Ⓖ ½ to ¾ cup (4 to 6 ounces)

1 In a small bowl, mix together the garlic powder, paprika, onion powder, thyme, black pepper, and sage.

2 Remove any giblets from the chicken cavity. Rinse the outside and inner cavity of the chicken under cold water and use a paper towel to pat dry. Place the chicken in the slow cooker.

3 Rub the chicken with the herb mixture, getting as much as possible under the skin.

4 Stuff the inside of the chicken with the rosemary and lemon wedges.

5 Cover the slow cooker and turn on low to cook for 7 hours, or until the temperature of the innermost part of a thigh and thickest part of the breast has reached 165°F.

Cooking tip: *Always practice good food-safety techniques when thawing raw meat, since it can be a source of harmful bacteria. Thaw it for 1 to 3 days in the fridge ahead of the day you desire to cook it. A more rapid method for thawing is using a cold water bath. Fill your sink or a very large stockpot with cold water, immerse the meat, and thaw for 2 to 3 hours, changing the water frequently to prevent the growth of harmful bacteria. Make sure to properly clean and sanitize your sink or pot after thawing.*

Per Serving (4 ounces): Calories: 191; Total fat: 8g; Protein: 29g; Carbs: 0g; Fiber: 0g; Sugar: 0g; Sodium: 86mg

Mediterranean Turkey Meatloaf

**SERVES 4 / PREP TIME: 10 MINUTES / COOK TIME: 55 MINUTES
TOTAL TIME: 65 MINUTES**

You've no doubt heard about the health benefits of following the Mediterranean diet. But how do you fit all of those foods into your new lifestyle when your sleeve can only accommodate such small portions? This meatloaf recipe is not the one your grandmother made—it's packed with Mediterranean-inspired ingredients, all mixed into a protein-packed meal. Try this tonight with a side of Baked Zucchini Fries (page 79).

For the meatloaf

Nonstick cooking spray

1 pound extra-lean ground turkey

1 large egg, lightly beaten

¼ cup whole-wheat bread crumbs

¼ fat-free feta cheese

¼ cup Kalamata olives, pitted and halved

¼ cup chopped fresh parsley

¼ cup minced red onion

¼ cup plus 2 tablespoons hummus, such as Lantana Cucumber Hummus, divided

2 teaspoons minced garlic

½ teaspoon dried basil

¼ teaspoon dried oregano

TO MAKE THE MEATLOAF

1 Preheat the oven to 350°F. Coat an 8-by-4-inch loaf pan with the cooking spray.

2 In a large bowl, combine the ground turkey, egg, bread crumbs, feta cheese, olives, parsley, onion, 2 tablespoons of hummus, garlic, basil, and oregano. Using clean hands, mix until just combined.

3 Place the meatloaf mixture evenly in the loaf pan. Spread the remaining ¼ cup of hummus over the top of the meatloaf.

4 Bake for 55 minutes.

For the topping

½ small cucumber, peeled, seeded, and chopped

1 large tomato, chopped

2 to 3 tablespoons minced fresh basil

Juice of ½ lemon

1 teaspoon extra-virgin olive oil

Post-Op Servings

S 2 ounces

G 2 to 4 ounces

TO MAKE THE TOPPING

1 In a small bowl, mix together the cucumber, tomato, basil, lemon juice, and olive oil. Refrigerate until ready to serve.

2 The meatloaf is done when it reaches an internal temperature of 165°F. Let it sit for 5 minutes before serving, then slice and garnish with the topping

Did You Know? *Olive oil is a super food with proven health benefits. Packed with monounsaturated fat, it has been shown to have beneficial effects on overall blood cholesterol levels when used in place of other saturated fats like butter or animal fats. The phytochemicals and polyphenols in olive oil may protect against cancer and provide other anti-inflammatory effects on the body. For the highest-quality version, choose extra-virgin, cold-pressed olive oil. Additionally, look for brands with the most recent harvested date. Some of the nutrients can be lost when left on the shelf for months at a time. Note that although olive oil is heart healthy, it contains the same amount of calories per teaspoon as butter or other fats, so keep portions moderate.*

Per Serving (4 ounces): Calories: 232; Total fat: 8g; Protein: 31g; Carbs: 10g; Fiber: 2g; Sugar: 2g; Sodium: 370mg

Mexican Taco Skillet with Red Peppers and Zucchini

**SERVES 6 / PREP TIME: 10 MINUTES / COOK TIME: 20 MINUTES
TOTAL TIME: 30 MINUTES**

When I ask patients what their go-to meals for the week include, tacos always seem to be on the menu. For the majority, it's the classic ground beef, cheese, and white tortilla shells. After gastric sleeve surgery, you may need to think twice about what you serve on your go-to taco night. Here is a one-pan meal you can substitute for traditional tacos that is just as quick and easy—and absolutely delicious.

2 teaspoons extra-virgin olive oil

1 large onion, finely chopped

1 tablespoon minced garlic

1 jalapeño pepper, seeded and finely chopped

2 medium red bell peppers, diced

1 pound boneless, skinless chicken breast, cut into 1-inch cubes

1 tablespoon ground cumin

1 teaspoon low-sodium taco seasoning, such as from Penzeys Spices

1 (14.5-ounce) can diced tomatoes

1 large zucchini, halved lengthwise and diced

½ cup shredded mild Cheddar cheese

1 cup chopped fresh cilantro

½ cup chopped scallions

1 In a large skillet over medium heat, heat the olive oil. Add the onion, garlic, jalapeño, and red bell peppers. Sauté the vegetables for about 5 minutes, or until tender.

2 Add the chicken, cumin, and taco seasoning, and stir until the chicken and vegetables are well coated.

3 Stir in the tomatoes. Bring the mixture to a boil. Cover the skillet, reduce the heat to medium-low, and cook for 10 minutes.

4 Add the zucchini and mix well. Cook for 7 minutes more, or until the zucchini is tender.

Post-Op Servings

 1 cup

5 Remove the skillet from the heat. Mix in the cheese, cilantro, and scallions, and serve.

Did You Know? *Bell peppers are an excellent source of vitamin C. This nutrient is important for its antioxidant and immune-boosting benefits. Choose bell peppers on a regular basis to get in this important vitamin and leave behind the commonly-consumed vitamin C-rich orange juice, which is high in sugar content.*

Per Serving (1 cup): Calories: 162; Total fat: 7g; Protein: 18g; Carbs: 8g; Fiber: 2g; Sugar: 5g; Sodium: 261mg

Cauliflower Pizza with Caramelized Onions and Chicken Sausage

MAKES 1 (12-INCH) PIZZA / PREP TIME: 20 MINUTES / COOK TIME: 35 MINUTES
TOTAL TIME: 55 MINUTES

Pizza is a staple in the typical American diet, and it's not a food that most people want to give up after weight-loss surgery. Fortunately, there are many ways to still enjoy pizza without the added carbs and fat. Many patients enjoy pizza by eating the toppings they scrape off the doughy crust—but still feel like they're missing out. Here's a low-carb version with a delicious cheesy cauliflower crust that will have you skipping delivery altogether and enjoying every bite guilt-free.

1 large head cauliflower, stemmed, with leaves removed

2 large eggs, lightly beaten

2 cups shredded part-skim mozzarella cheese, divided

½ cup shredded Parmigiano-Reggiano cheese

½ teaspoon dried oregano

¼ teaspoon dried basil

½ teaspoon garlic powder

2 teaspoons extra-virgin olive oil

2 red onions, thinly sliced

2 links precooked chicken sausage (nitrate-free), cut into ¼-inch rounds

Post-Op Servings

Ⓖ 1 or 2 slices

1 Preheat the oven to 400°F.

2 Cut the cauliflower head into 3 or 4 large pieces. Place in a food processor and pulse for 1 to 2 seconds at a time until all the pieces are the size of rice. Remove any large pieces that won't break down. Transfer the riced cauliflower to a bowl and pat dry with a paper towel.

3 Place a small pot over medium heat and add ½ cup water. Put the riced cauliflower directly in the pot (or in a steamer basket in the pot), and bring the water to a boil. Cover the pot and steam the cauliflower for 3 to 5 minutes, or until tender. Remove the pan from the heat and let cool. Place the steamed cauliflower on a paper towel to soak up any moisture and pat dry.

4 In a medium bowl, combine the eggs, 1 cup of mozzarella, Parmigiano-Reggiano cheese, oregano, basil, and garlic powder. Add the cauliflower and mix well.

5 Spread the cauliflower mixture onto a 12-inch round pizza pan, and press it into an even layer like a pizza crust. Press until it is less than 1-inch thick. Bake for 20 minutes.

6 While the crust bakes, place a large skillet over medium heat. Heat the olive oil and add the onions and cook, stirring occasionally, until caramelized, about 20 minutes.

7 Spread the caramelized onions and chicken sausage evenly across the cauliflower crust. Top with the remaining 1 cup of mozzarella cheese. Bake the pizza for 10 minutes more, or until the cheese is bubbly.

Cooking tip: *Make your own frozen pizza. Batch cook several pizza crusts and top with your favorite toppings. Wrap securely in plastic wrap and aluminum foil and toss in the freezer. When you want to use it, unwrap it, and place the pizza in a preheated oven for 20 minutes for a quick weeknight meal.*

Per Serving (1 slice): Calories: 121; Total fat: 7g; Protein: 10g; Carbs: 8g; Fiber: 4g; Sugar: 3g; Sodium: 260mg

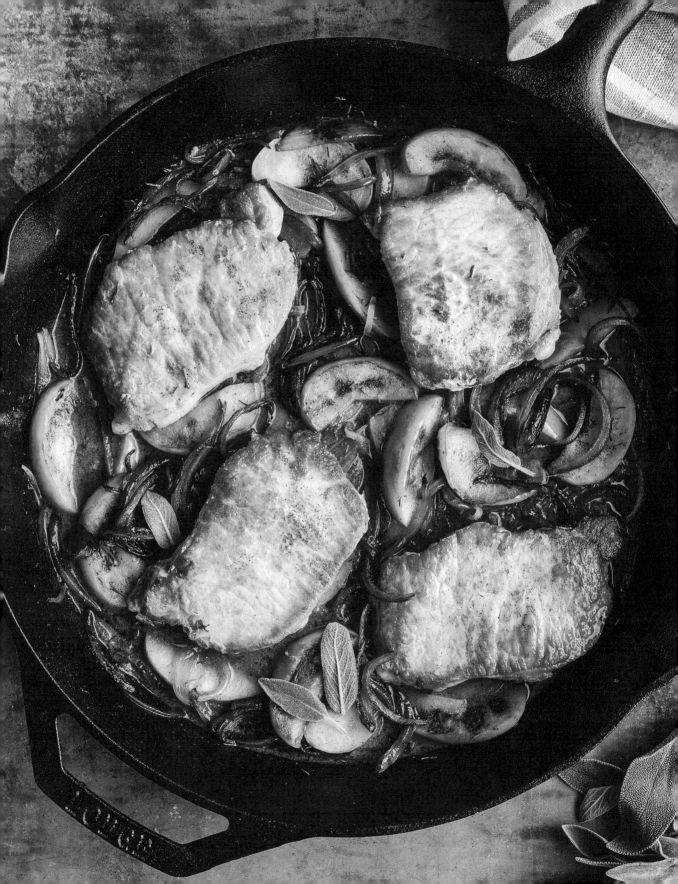

CHAPTER NINE

Pork and Beef Dinners

Chipotle Shredded Pork

SERVES 8 / PREP TIME: 10 MINUTES / COOK TIME: 6 HOURS
TOTAL TIME: 6 HOURS, 10 MINUTES

Try this slow-cooked smoky, spicy, pulled pork, which takes an otherwise tough cut of meat and makes it oh-so-tender—and thus a perfect recipe for the VSG Club. Better still, it's a simple recipe for even the most novice chef. You can toss this together on the weekend to put in the slow cooker on Monday or Tuesday for a quick weeknight meal. Serve inside low-carb taco shells for carnitas, on a low-calorie whole-wheat bun for sandwiches (try topped with a Greek yogurt–based coleslaw), or serve alongside a cup of Baked Potato Soup (page 120).

1 (7.5-ounce) can chipotle peppers in adobo sauce

1½ tablespoons apple cider vinegar

1 tablespoon ground cumin

1 tablespoon dried oregano

Juice of 1 lime

2 pounds pork shoulder, trimmed of excess fat

Post-Op Servings

 ½ cup pork

1 In a blender or food processor, puree the chipotle peppers and adobo sauce, apple cider vinegar, cumin, oregano, and lime juice.

2 Place the pork shoulder in the slow cooker, and pour the sauce over it.

3 Cover the slow cooker, and cook on low for 6 hours.

4 The finished pork should shred easily. Use two forks to shred the pork in the slow cooker. If there is any additional sauce, allow the pork to cook on low for 20 minutes more to absorb the remaining liquid.

Post-op tip: *Variety is the spice of life, but is it the best method for weight loss? Sometimes having similar types of meals on a daily basis, such as the same breakfast or lunch, can help limit the guesswork and keep calories or portions controlled. Although it's important to get a variety of nutrients in your diet—it's A-OK to use a simple meal plan to keep yourself on track!*

Per Serving (½ cup pork): Calories: 260; Total fat: 11g; Protein: 20g; Carbs: 5g; Fiber: 2g; Sugar: 2g; Sodium: 705mg

One-Pan Pork Chops with Apples and Red Onion

SERVES 4 / PREP TIME: 10 MINUTES / COOK TIME: 30 MINUTES
TOTAL TIME: 40 MINUTES

These pork chops are flavorful and melt-in-your-mouth tender. The sweet cooked apples are a perfect balance for the savory pork—that's why it's a classic combination. Plus, you can keep a clean kitchen by using just one pot. Try serving with Roasted Root Vegetables (page 84) as a side dish or over Cauliflower Rice (page 85).

2 teaspoons extra-virgin olive oil, divided

4 boneless center-cut thin pork chops

2 small apples, thinly sliced

1 small red onion, thinly sliced

1 cup low-sodium chicken broth

1 teaspoon Dijon mustard

1 teaspoon dried sage

1 teaspoon dried thyme

Post-Op Servings

Ⓖ ½ to 1 pork chop

1 Place a large nonstick frying pan over high heat and add 1 teaspoon of olive oil. When the oil is hot, add the pork chops and reduce the heat to medium. Sear the chops for 3 minutes on one side, flip, and sear the other side for 3 minutes, 6 minutes total. Transfer the chops to a plate and set aside.

2 In the same pan, add the remaining 1 teaspoon of olive oil. Add the apples and onion. Cook for 5 minutes or until tender, stirring frequently to prevent burning.

3 While the apples and onion cook, mix together the broth and Dijon mustard in a small bowl.

4 Add the sage and thyme to the pan and stir to coat the onion and apples. Stir in the broth mixture and return the pork chops to the pan. Cover the pan and simmer for 10 to 15 minutes.

5 Let pork chops rest for 2 minutes before cutting.

Per Serving (1 pork chop): Calories: 234; Total fat: 11g; Protein: 20g; Carbs: 13g; Fiber: 3g; Sugar: 9g; Sodium: 290mg

Slow Cooker Pork with Red Peppers and Pineapple

SERVES 4 / PREP TIME: 10 MINUTES / COOK TIME: 5 HOURS / TOTAL TIME: 5 HOURS, 10 MINUTES

Depending on how it's prepared, pork can be a tough meat. With a smaller stomach after the sleeve gastrectomy, you might have a harder time digesting dense foods. This slow-cooked pork is naturally tenderized by the enzymes in the pineapple. I recommend using canned pineapple since it seems to be less fibrous than fresh. Serve the pork by itself or over Cauliflower Rice (page 85). This meal freezes well and stays moist when reheated.

¼ cup low-sodium soy sauce or Bragg Liquid Aminos

Juice of ½ lemon

1 teaspoon garlic powder

1 teaspoon ground cumin

½ teaspoon cayenne pepper

¼ teaspoon ground coriander

1½ pounds boneless pork tenderloin

2 red bell peppers, thinly sliced

2 (20-ounce) cans pineapple chunks in 100% natural juice or water, drained

Post-Op Servings

Ⓖ 2 to 4 ounces

1 In a small bowl, mix together the soy sauce, lemon juice, garlic powder, cumin, cayenne pepper, and coriander.

2 Place the pork tenderloin in the slow cooker and add the red bell pepper slices. Cover with the pineapple chunks and their juices. Pour the soy sauce mixture on top.

3 Cover the slow cooker and turn on low for about 5 hours.

4 Shred the pork with a fork and tongs and continue to cook on low for 20 minutes more, or until juices are absorbed.

5 Serve and enjoy!

Ingredient tip: *If you're not familiar with Bragg Liquid Aminos, it is a liquid protein concentrate, derived from soybeans. It contains all 16 amino acids and has a taste that's very similar to soy sauce.*

Per Serving (3 ounces): Calories: 131; Total fat: 2g; Protein: 17g; Carbs: 11g; Fiber: 2g; Sugar: 8g; Sodium: 431mg

Pork, White Bean, and Spinach Soup

SERVES 4 TO 6 / PREP TIME: 10 MINUTES / COOK TIME: 40 MINUTES
TOTAL TIME: 50 MINUTES

Pork and beans just seem to go well together. This soup pairs the rich, smoky flavor of pork with savory spinach and white beans. It's a simple recipe to toss together on a weeknight. Sear the pork before making the rest of the soup to lock in the juices and to keep the meat tender.

1 teaspoon extra-virgin olive oil

1 medium onion, chopped

2 (4-ounce) boneless pork chops, cut into 1-inch cubes

1 (14.5 ounce) can diced tomatoes

3 cups low-sodium chicken broth

½ teaspoon dried thyme

¼ teaspoon crushed red pepper flakes

1 (15-ounce) can great northern beans, drained and rinsed

8 ounces fresh spinach leaves

Post-Op Servings

G 1 cup

1 Place a large soup pot or Dutch oven over medium heat and heat the olive oil.

2 Add the onion and sauté for 2 to 3 minutes, or until tender. Add the pork and brown it for 4 to 5 minutes on each side.

3 Mix in the tomatoes, broth, thyme, red pepper flakes, and beans. Bring to a boil and then reduce the heat to low to simmer, covered, for 30 minutes.

4 Add the spinach and stir until wilted, about 5 minutes, and serve immediately.

Did You Know? *Pork (and all meats, eggs, and dairy) is an excellent source of vitamin B_{12}, which is important for preventing anemia and is crucial for nerve function. Because of changes in the absorption of vitamin B_{12} and a risk of its deficiency after bariatric surgery, many patients need a B_{12} supplement in the form of a pill or injection. Eating foods that are high in vitamin B_{12} is a good way to keep those levels topped up.*

Per Serving (1 cup): Calories: 156; Total fat: 4g; Protein: 17g; Carbs: 17g; Fiber: 4g; Sugar: 6g; Sodium: 600mg

Beef Stew with Rutabaga and Carrots

SERVES 6 / PREP TIME: 15 MINUTES / COOK TIME: 40 MINUTES
TOTAL TIME: 55 MINUTES

One-pot meals are a great way to get both protein and vegetables without a lot of hassle or dirty dishes. This beef stew recipe is super flavorful and foolproof. The unique flavor of the rutabaga balances out the richness of the meat. Rutabaga is a great source of fiber, vitamin C, and potassium. It's a cruciferous vegetable, so it offers some of the same health benefits as broccoli, cauliflower, and cabbage, including fighting cancer. This meal freezes well and serves up nicely as leftovers to save on meal preparation for lunches or dinners later in the week.

4 teaspoons extra-virgin olive oil, divided

1 pound beef sirloin steak, cut into 1-inch cubes

2 teaspoons minced garlic

1 medium onion, chopped

1 pound rutabaga, peeled, and cut into ½-inch cubes

3 medium carrots, peeled, and cut into ½-inch cubes

1 small tomato, diced

1 teaspoon smoked paprika

½ teaspoon ground coriander

¼ teaspoon red pepper flakes

2 tablespoons whole-wheat flour

½ cup red wine

3 cups low-sodium beef broth

Fresh minced parsley, for garnish

1 In a large soup pot or Dutch oven, heat 2 teaspoons of olive oil over medium heat.

2 Add the beef and brown it on all sides, stirring frequently, until no longer pink, about 5 minutes. Transfer to a bowl and set aside.

3 In the same pot, heat the remaining 2 teaspoons of olive oil over medium heat. Add the garlic and onion, and cook, stirring frequently, until the onion is tender, 1 to 2 minutes.

4 Stir in the rutabaga, carrots, tomato, paprika, coriander, and red pepper flakes.

5 Add the flour and cook, stirring constantly, for 1 minute. Add the red wine and stir for an additional minute.

Post-Op Servings

 1 cup

6 Add the broth and return the beef to the pot. Bring to a boil and then reduce the heat to low to simmer. The sauce should start to thicken. Cover the pot and cook for 30 minutes, or until all the vegetables are tender.

7 Serve garnished with the parsley.

Cooking tip: *Don't waste the leftover wine from your last dinner party! Keep both red and white wine leftovers to use in cooking. They add a unique flavor and can be a replacement for broth. Steer clear of purchasing cooking wine that contains lots of added sodium. You can swap in red wine for beef broth or white wine for chicken broth. Don't worry about the alcohol content, as it will cook off when simmered.*

Per Serving (1 cup): Calories: 224; Total Fat: 10g; Protein: 17g; Carbs: 13g; Fiber: 3g; Sugars: 5g; Sodium: 139 mg

Spaghetti Squash Casserole with Ground Beef

SERVES 8 / PREP TIME: 10 MINUTES / COOK TIME: 75 MINUTES
TOTAL TIME: 1 HOUR, 25 MINUTES

Nothing like a dish of spaghetti with beef sauce to fill an empty stomach after a long day of work. Just because you can't have starchy pasta doesn't mean you can't have a meal just as comforting, with cheese and beef and only one-third of the carbs. Prepare to be satisfied with loads of ooey-gooey cheese and beefy goodness as you swap pasta for spaghetti squash in this casserole recipe.

Nonstick cooking spray

2 medium spaghetti squash (2½ to 3 pounds)

1 pound supreme lean ground beef

1 large onion, minced

2 teaspoons minced garlic

1 (8-ounce) can tomato sauce

1 (10-ounce) can diced tomatoes

1 teaspoon dried basil

1 teaspoon dried oregano

1 cup shredded mozzarella cheese

½ cup shredded Parmigiano-Reggiano cheese

Post-Op Servings

 1 cup serving

1 Preheat the oven to 350°F. Coat a baking sheet with the cooking spray.

2 Halve the spaghetti squash, remove and discard the stem, pulp, and seeds, and place the halves cut-side down on the baking sheet. Bake for about 35 minutes, or until the flesh is tender.

3 While the squash bakes, spray a large skillet with the cooking spray, and place it over medium heat. Add the ground beef, onion, and garlic, and sauté for about 10 minutes, or until the beef is no longer pink and the onion is tender. Add the tomato sauce, diced tomatoes, basil, and oregano and stir to combine well. Remove the pan from the heat and set aside.

4 When the spaghetti squash is cool enough to handle, carefully use a fork to pull the flesh from the outer skin and make "spaghetti." Set aside in a bowl.

5 In a 9-by-13-inch baking dish, layer one-third of the meat-and-tomato mixture in the bottom of the dish. Evenly spread half of the squash over the meat layer. Layer another one-third of the meat mixture over the squash. Finish the last layer with the second half of the squash and the last one-third of the meat mixture. Sprinkle the mozzarella and Parmigiano-Reggiano cheeses over the top.

6 Cover with aluminum foil and bake for 30 minutes. Remove the foil and bake for 10 minutes more, or until the cheese begins to brown. Serve.

Cooking tip: *Going vegetarian? Replace the beef in this recipe with ground soybeans or another vegetarian ground beef alternative. Add an additional 1/2 cup water to the "meat"-and-tomato mixture to keep it moist.*

Per Serving (1 cup): Calories: 229; Total fat: 10g; Protein: 20g; Carbs: 16g; Fiber: 3g; Sugar: 11g; Sodium: 511mg

Italian Beef Sandwiches

MAKES 6 SANDWICHES / PREP TIME: 10 MINUTES / COOK TIME: 7 HOURS
TOTAL TIME: 7 HOURS, 10 MINUTES

Before weight-loss surgery you may have enjoyed the occasional beef sandwich laden with sauce and served on a doughy bun. This is a fantastic recipe for a slow-cooked beef sandwich, but with a healthy twist. Using a slow cooker to prepare beef helps get the perfect texture for when you add more red meat back to your diet. For hot dog buns, I recommend Angelic Bakehouse.

1 cup water

1 tablespoon
balsamic vinegar

¾ teaspoon garlic powder

¾ teaspoon onion powder

1½ teaspoons
dried parsley

¾ teaspoon dried oregano

¼ teaspoon dried thyme

½ teaspoon dried basil

¼ teaspoon freshly
ground black pepper

1½ pounds boneless beef
chuck roast,
fat trimmed

1 medium onion, sliced

1 red bell pepper, cut
into strips

6 sprouted-grain hot dog
buns or sandwich thins

1 (16-ounce) jar
pepperoncini (optional)

1 In a small bowl mix together the water, balsamic vinegar, garlic powder, onion powder, parsley, oregano, thyme, basil, and black pepper.

2 Place the beef in the slow cooker and add the onion and bell pepper.

3 Pour the sauce over the roast. Cover the slow cooker and cook on low for 7 hours. The meat should be tender and cooked through.

4 Carefully transfer the roast to a cutting board.

5 Thinly slice the roast.

Post-Op Servings

 1 sandwich

6 Toast the buns or sandwich thins.

7 Layer each bun with the beef and top with the au jus, pepper, and onion. Serve with pepperoncini (if using).

Post-op tip: *A word about starches: Doughy bread products are not well tolerated after weight-loss surgery and should be avoided to help keep carbohydrate counts down. Most people find that eventually they can tolerate toasted bread products—but the thinner, the better (no large deli rolls). For this recipe you may decide to forgo the bun altogether and serve up the meat with vegetables, or you may try just half of a bun. Always focus on eating protein first before filling up on carbohydrates.*

Per Serving (1 sandwich): Calories: 351; Total fat: 9g; Protein: 31g; Carbs: 30g; Fiber: 5g; Sugar: 5g; Sodium: 418mg

Mom's Sloppy Joes

SERVES 8 / PREP TIME: 10 MINUTES / COOK TIME: 30 MINUTES
TOTAL TIME: 40 MINUTES

Revisit your childhood and enjoy this American classic made with wholesome ingredients, more flavors, and less salt than the premade canned versions. This recipe takes me back to memories of quick weeknight meals when my mother was trying to feed four kids in a hurry and on a budget—plus serve us something we actually liked! These sloppy joes have so much flavor you can eat them without any bun to keep the carbohydrates down.

Nonstick cooking spray

1½ pounds supreme lean ground beef

1 cup chopped onion

1 cup chopped celery

1 (8-ounce) can tomato sauce

⅓ cup catsup (free of high-fructose corn syrup)

2 tablespoons white vinegar

2 tablespoons Worcestershire sauce

2 tablespoons Dijon mustard

1 tablespoon brown sugar

Post-Op Servings

Ⓖ ¾ cup sloppy joe

1 Spray a large skillet with the cooking spray, and place it over medium heat. Add the beef and brown until it is no longer pink, about 10 minutes. Drain off any grease.

2 Mix in the onion and celery, and cook for 2 to 3 minutes.

3 Stir in the tomato sauce, catsup, vinegar, Worcestershire sauce, mustard, and brown sugar. Bring the liquid to a simmer, and reduce the heat to low. Cook for 15 minutes, or until the sauce has thickened.

4 Spoon about ¾ cup of the sloppy joe mixture onto each plate, and serve.

Serving tip: *If you can tolerate bread, try these sloppy joes served open-faced on half of a toasted thin roll, such as Thomas' 100% whole-grain sandwich thins.*

Per Serving (¾ cup): Calories: 269; Total fat: 5g; Protein: 24g; Carbs: 32g; Fiber: 6g; Sugar: 6g; Sodium: 656mg

Creamy Beef Stroganoff with Mushrooms

MAKES 6 SERVINGS / PREP TIME: 10 MINUTES / COOK TIME: 30 MINUTES
TOTAL TIME: 40 MINUTES

There's nothing more filling than wholesome beef Stroganoff to fill you up when you're feeling hungry, but the combination of high-fat creamy sauce and rich beef in traditional recipes won't agree with your sleeve after surgery. Try this healthier twist on the traditional recipe made with simple staple ingredients from your kitchen. Serve over zucchini noodles or Cauliflower Rice (page 85) instead of pasta to keep carbohydrate servings in check.

Nonstick cooking spray

1½ pounds extra-lean beef sirloin, cut into ½-inch strips

1 teaspoon extra-virgin olive oil

1 medium onion, chopped

½ pound mushrooms, sliced

2 tablespoon whole-wheat flour

1 cup low-sodium beef broth

1 cup water

1 teaspoon Worcestershire sauce

½ teaspoon dried thyme

½ teaspoon dried dill

½ cup low-fat plain Greek yogurt

2 tablespoons finely chopped fresh parsley, for garnish

Post-Op Servings

G 4 ounces

1 Coat a medium pan with the cooking spray and place over medium-high heat. Add the beef. Cook, stirring frequently, until browned, about 5 minutes. Transfer to a bowl and set aside.

2 In the same pan, heat the olive oil over medium-high heat. Add the onion and cook until tender, 1 to 2 minutes.

3 Add the mushrooms and cook until tender, about 3 minutes.

4 Mix in the flour and stir to coat the onion and mushrooms.

5 Stir in the broth, water, Worcestershire sauce, thyme, dill. Bring to a boil, cover the pan, and cook for about 10 minutes, stirring frequently.

6 Stir in the yogurt. Mix in the beef. Serve, garnished with the parsley.

Per Serving (4 ounces): Calories: 351; Total fat: 9g; Protein: 31g; Carbs: 30g; Fiber: 5g; Sugar: 5g; Sodium: 418mg

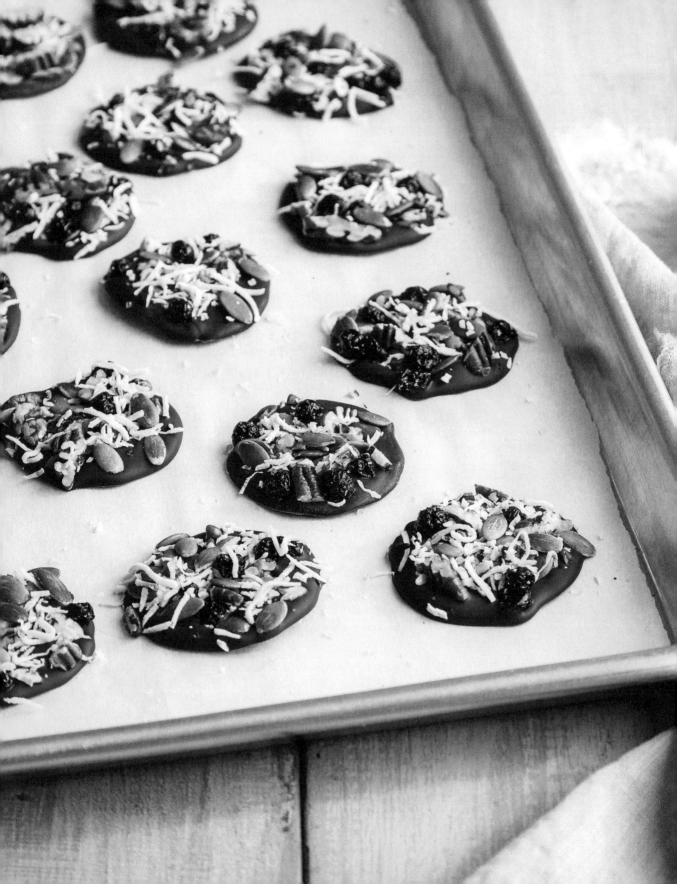

CHAPTER TEN

Sweets and Treats

Superfood Dark Chocolates

MAKES 18 CHOCOLATES / PREP TIME: 5 MINUTES / COOK TIME: 25 MINUTES
TOTAL TIME: 30 MINUTES

When it comes to dessert after bariatric surgery, sweets should be avoided whenever possible to keep calories controlled and maximize weight loss. With that in mind, if and when you do indulge, go for something high quality to make it worthwhile, but keep sugars to a minimum to prevent any unforeseen side effects from consuming too much. I love these little homemade chocolates because they are packed with nutrient-rich ingredients and made with heart-healthy antioxidant-rich dark chocolate. Serve these at your next dinner party and you will impress your guests. You can even make these ahead of time and freeze them.

6 ounces dark chocolate chips (60% cacao or higher, such as Ghirardelli dark chocolate chips)

¼ cup pumpkin seeds (pepitas), chopped

¼ cup unsweetened shredded coconut

¼ cup chopped pecans

¼ cup unsweetened dried wild blueberries

1 teaspoon sea salt

Post-Op Servings

 1 chocolate

1 Line 1 or 2 baking sheets with parchment paper.

2 Fill a large pot with water and bring it to a boil. Reduce the heat to a simmer and place a stainless steel heat-proof bowl over the top of the boiling water. Add the chocolate chips and stir until melted and smooth. Alternatively, you can use a double boiler or melt the chocolate in the microwave (use 50 percent power and stir frequently to prevent burning).

3 Use a spoon to drizzle the melted chocolate on the sheet pan in small circles (about ¾ tablespoon of chocolate in circles about 2 inches in diameter).

4 Add the pumpkin seeds, coconut, pecans, and dried blueberries to each chocolate circle. Each should hold about ¾ tablespoon of toppings total. Sprinkle with the sea salt.

5 Let the chocolates harden at room temperature or in the refrigerator. Keep them in an airtight container and eat within 2 weeks to maintain maximum freshness.

Serving tip: *Get creative with your superfood toppings. Add chia seeds for crunch and added fiber; use other dried fruits like sliced figs, cranberries, or mango; or swap in other nuts like chopped cashews or shelled pistachios. Portion control is key, though, as dried fruits often contain added sugars and they're dense in calories.*

Per Serving (1 chocolate): Calories: 102; Total fat: 7g; Protein: 3g; Carbs: 8g; Fiber: 2g; Sugar: 6g; Sodium: 99mg

Chocolate Chia Pudding

SERVES 4 / PREP TIME: 15 MINUTES, PLUS 60 MINUTES TO CHILL
TOTAL TIME: 1 HOUR, 15 MINUTES

Try this recipe for a new take on pudding. The chia seeds thicken the milk and create the perfect creamy texture without using any gelatin or other additives. Plus, chia seeds are loaded with fiber and omega-3 fats, so just a taste will keep you full and satisfied. This recipe uses unsweetened cocoa, which provides all the chocolate goodness without all the sugar.

2 cups unsweetened soy milk

10 drops liquid stevia

¼ cup unsweetened cocoa powder

¼ teaspoon ground cinnamon

¼ teaspoon vanilla extract

½ cup chia seeds

½ cup fresh raspberries, for garnish

1 In a small bowl, whisk together the soy milk, stevia, cocoa powder, cinnamon, and vanilla until well combined.

2 Stir in the chia seeds.

3 Divide between 4 small serving dishes.

4 Cover and refrigerate for at least 1 hour, or overnight.

5 When ready to serve, garnish with the raspberries.

Post-Op Servings

 ½ cup

Ingredient tip: *Chia seeds form a gelatinous texture when mixed with water. They can be used in baking to replace other ingredients to add calcium and fiber with no cholesterol. Make chia gel by mixing 1 tablespoon of chia seeds with 6 tablespoons of water. Let sit for 30 minutes. Use ¼ cup of chia gel to replace an egg or swap for one-quarter of cooking oil in baking recipes.*

Per Serving (½ cup): Calories 182; Total fat: 9g; Protein: 11g; Carbs: 14g; Fiber: 14g; Sugars: 1g; Sodium: 36mg

Easy Peanut Butter Cookies

MAKES 15 COOKIES / PREP TIME: 15 MINUTES / COOK TIME: 15 MINUTES
TOTAL TIME: 30 MINUTES

Sometimes you need a sweet treat and you don't have a lot of time to mix together a long list of ingredients. These easy four-ingredient peanut butter cookies are low in sugar since they're made with stevia, but so tasty they will certainly satisfy your sweet tooth.

Nonstick cooking spray
1 cup natural smooth peanut butter
1 large egg
½ cup stevia baking blend
½ teaspoon vanilla extract

Post-Op Servings

 1 cookie

1 Preheat the oven to 350°F. Coat a nonstick baking sheet with the cooking spray or use parchment paper.

2 In a medium bowl, use a hand mixer to combine the peanut butter, egg, stevia, and vanilla.

3 Roll the batter into 1-inch balls and place them on the baking sheet. Flatten each ball to about ¼-inch thickness. Using a fork, create two imprints of a crisscross pattern on the cookie.

4 Bake for about 12 minutes. The cookies are done when golden brown.

5 Cool for 5 minutes, then move to a baking rack to finish cooling.

Ingredient tip: *Peanut butter is dense in calories and fat—but it's loaded with good-for-you and heart-healthy monounsaturated fat. Choose natural versions that require you to mix the oil and peanut paste together. Stay away from any versions that include partially hydrogenated oils (trans fats) or palm oil (saturated fat). Many commercial versions in which the peanuts and oil are already mixed together also contain added sugars. Stick to the cleaner version and enjoy in moderate portions to keep calories in check.*

Per Serving (1 cookie): Calories: 107; Total fat: 9g; Protein: 4g; Carbs: 4g; Fiber: 1g; Sugar: 2g; Sodium: 47mg

Chocolate Brownies with Almond Butter

MAKES 16 BROWNIES / PREP TIME: 5 MINUTES / COOK TIME: 25 MINUTES
TOTAL TIME: 30 MINUTES

Make cocoa powder a pantry staple. It will give you the chocolate flavor without all the fat, sugar, and calories of traditional milk chocolate. These chocolate brownies have all the fudgy texture of a boxed mix but are made with healthy fat and agave nectar. Although agave is a sugar, it has a lower glycemic index than white sugar and may raise the blood sugar more gradually. If you don't like almond butter, feel free to replace it with smooth peanut butter.

Nonstick cooking spray
½ cup cocoa powder
1 tablespoon ground flaxseed
½ teaspoon ground instant coffee
¼ teaspoon baking soda
½ cup almond butter
¼ cup melted coconut oil
2 large eggs
1 teaspoon vanilla extract
½ cup agave nectar

Post-Op Servings

Ⓖ 1 brownie

1 Preheat the oven to 325°F. Coat an 8-by-8-inch glass baking dish with the cooking spray.

2 Place the cocoa powder, flaxseed, instant coffee, baking soda, almond butter, coconut oil, eggs, vanilla, and agave nectar in a high-speed blender or food processor. Blend on medium-high until smooth. Pour the batter into the baking dish.

3 Bake for 25 minutes or until a toothpick inserted in the middle comes out clean. Let cool for 10 minutes before cutting into 16 squares.

Serving tip: *Allowing dessert but concerned about overdoing the servings? Portion out the brownies and freeze them in freezer-safe resealable bags or containers. Thaw one serving at a time to allow yourself an occasional treat.*

Per Serving (1 brownie): Calories: 124; Total fat: 9g; Protein: 3g; Carbs: 11g; Fiber: 2g; Sugar: 9g; Sodium: 49mg

Lemon-Blackberry Frozen Yogurt

MAKES 4 CUPS / PREP TIME: 10 MINUTES / TOTAL TIME: 10 MINUTES

Cool and creamy ice cream and frozen yogurt go hand in hand with the hot days of summer. While your previous iced favorites might be off limits after weight-loss surgery, this frozen yogurt will satisfy your urge for ice cream. It takes just four ingredients and can be made in less than 10 minutes, which means you can enjoy this dessert all summer long.

4 cups frozen blackberries
½ cup low-fat plain
    Greek yogurt
Juice of 1 lemon
2 teaspoons liquid stevia
Fresh mint leaves,
    for garnish

Post-Op Servings

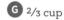 2/3 cup

1 In a blender or food processor, add the blackberries, yogurt, lemon juice, and stevia. Blend until smooth, about 5 minutes.

2 Serve immediately or freeze in an airtight container and use within 3 weeks. Garnish with fresh mint leaves.

Serving tip: *Get creative and mix and match unique flavors for your fro-yo. Use flavored Greek yogurt (low-sugar versions, if possible) as a base, and mix and match other fruits and herbs to switch it up! Try watermelon with lime and cayenne pepper or coconut with mango.*

Per Serving (⅔ cup): Calories: 68; Total fat: 0g; Protein: 3g; Total Carb: 15g; Fiber: 5g; Sugar: 11g; Sodium: 12mg

Old-Fashioned Apple Crisp

SERVES 10 / PREP TIME: 15 MINUTES / COOK TIME: 45 MINUTES
TOTAL TIME: 1 HOUR

Just because you won't be baking many pies after the sleeve gastrectomy doesn't mean you have to deny yourself the delights of fruit-based desserts. This apple crisp contains whole, fresh apples topped with heart-healthy oatmeal and sweetened with calorie-free stevia. I recommend baking this just before having guests over, as the whole house will smell sweet and delicious!

Nonstick cooking spray

6 apples, cored, peeled, and cut into 1-inch chunks

½ cup water

3 teaspoons stevia powder, divided

1 tablespoon cornstarch

½ teaspoon ground cinnamon

¼ teaspoon ground nutmeg

Juice of ½ lemon

¾ cup old-fashioned oats

¾ cup whole-wheat pastry flour

½ cup low-fat plain Greek yogurt

¼ cup coconut oil, melted

Post-Op Servings

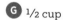 **G** ½ cup

1 Preheat the oven to 350°F. Coat an 8-by-8-inch baking dish with the cooking spray.

2 Put the apples, water, 1½ teaspoons of stevia, cornstarch, cinnamon, nutmeg, and lemon juice in the baking dish. Mix together. Bake for 20 minutes.

3 Meanwhile, in a medium bowl, combine the oats, flour, and the remaining 1½ teaspoons of stevia. Mix in the yogurt and coconut oil. Stir until all the flour is mixed and moistened throughout.

4 Evenly cover the apple mixture with the oatmeal mixture. Bake for 25 minutes more, or until the topping is golden brown.

5 Serve immediately.

Cooking tip: *Baking or grilling fruit brings out its natural sweetness. Try alternative versions of fruit crisp made with cherries, peaches, or pears.*

Per Serving (½ cup): Calories: 170; Total fat: 6g; Protein: 3g; Carbs: 28g; Fiber: 5g; Sugar: 8g; Sodium: 7mg

No-Bake Peanut Butter Protein Bites with Dark Chocolate

MAKES 25 BITES / PREP TIME: 20 MINUTES, PLUS 30 MINUTES TO CHILL
TOTAL TIME: 50 MINUTES

Energy bites, superfood balls, power squares . . . these little nutrient-packed snacks can be found lining the shelves of your health food and grocery stores for a high price. Make them at home for less money and an even better taste. These protein bites are packed with energy in the form of nutrient-dense ingredients and calories, so portion control is an absolute must. But with a great combination of carbohydrates, fat, and protein, they are an excellent pre- or post-workout snack—bring them along for your next hiking adventure!

1 cup old-fashioned rolled oats

1 cup vanilla protein powder

¾ cup smooth natural peanut butter

2 tablespoons ground flaxseed

1 tablespoon chia seeds

1 teaspoon vanilla extract

¼ cup dark chocolate chips

¾ teaspoon stevia baking blend

1 tablespoon water (or more or less to reach desired consistency)

1 Mix together the oats, protein powder, peanut butter, flaxseed, chia seeds, vanilla, chocolate chips, stevia, and water in a large mixing bowl.

2 Refrigerate for at least 30 minutes.

3 Roll into 25 balls. Store in an airtight container in the refrigerator.

4 Eat within 1 week or freeze.

Cooking tip: *Mix and match the dry or wet ingredients to make simple swaps. Add coconut and cocoa powder for a chocolate fix, or try sunflower seed butter instead of peanut butter to go nut-free. You can also add some pumpkin puree and cinnamon for a fall treat.*

Post-Op Servings

 1 to 2 bites

Per Serving (2 bites): Calories: 181; Total fat: 10g; Protein: 11g; Carbs: 11g; Fiber: 3g; Sugar: 3g; Sodium: 105mg

Low-Carb Crustless Cherry Cheesecake

SERVES 10 / PREP TIME: 10 MINUTES / COOK TIME: 45 MINUTES, PLUS 2 HOURS TO CHILL / TOTAL TIME: LESS THAN 3 HOURS

I'm always on the lookout for great, crowd-pleasing desserts that don't have all the added sugar and fat. I hit the jackpot with this creamy cheesecake recipe. It's a melt-in-your-mouth cheesecake topped with sweet and tart cherries. Enjoy this recipe guilt-free after surgery.

For the cheesecake

Nonstick cooking spray

2 (8-ounce) packages Neufchâtel cheese, at room temperature

Juice of ½ lemon

¼ cup nonfat plain Greek yogurt

2 teaspoons vanilla extract

¼ cup stevia baking blend

3 large eggs

For the topping

12 ounces frozen cherries, stemmed and pitted

2 tablespoons water

2 teaspoons cornstarch

1 teaspoon stevia baking blend

Post-Op Servings

Ⓖ 1 piece (¹⁄₁₀th cheesecake) with cherry topping

TO MAKE THE CHEESECAKE

1 Preheat the oven to 325°F. Coat a 9-inch springform pan or pie plate with the cooking spray.

2 In a large bowl, mix together the Neufchâtel cheese, lemon juice, yogurt, and vanilla.

3 Add the stevia and mix until smooth.

4 Next mix in the eggs, one at a time, until well blended. Pour the filling into the pan.

5 Bake for 35 to 45 minutes, or until the center is set. When done, the cheesecake should be slightly browned and barely firm in center.

1 While the cheesecake bakes, place a medium pot over medium-high heat. Put the cherries and water in the pot and bring to a boil, then reduce the heat to medium-low. Simmer until the cherries begin to bubble.

2 Stir 2 tablespoons of the cherry juices into the cornstarch. Stir this slurry into the cherries. This will thicken the topping. Stir in the stevia. Remove the pot from the heat and set aside to cool.

3 Cool the cheesecake for 30 minutes before refrigerating. Refrigerate for at least 2 hours, or overnight, before serving.

4 Serve with the cherry topping.

Per Serving (1 piece with cherry topping): Calories: 156; Total fat: 10g; Protein: 6g; Carbs: 7g; Fiber: 1g; Sugar: 5g; Sodium: 215mg

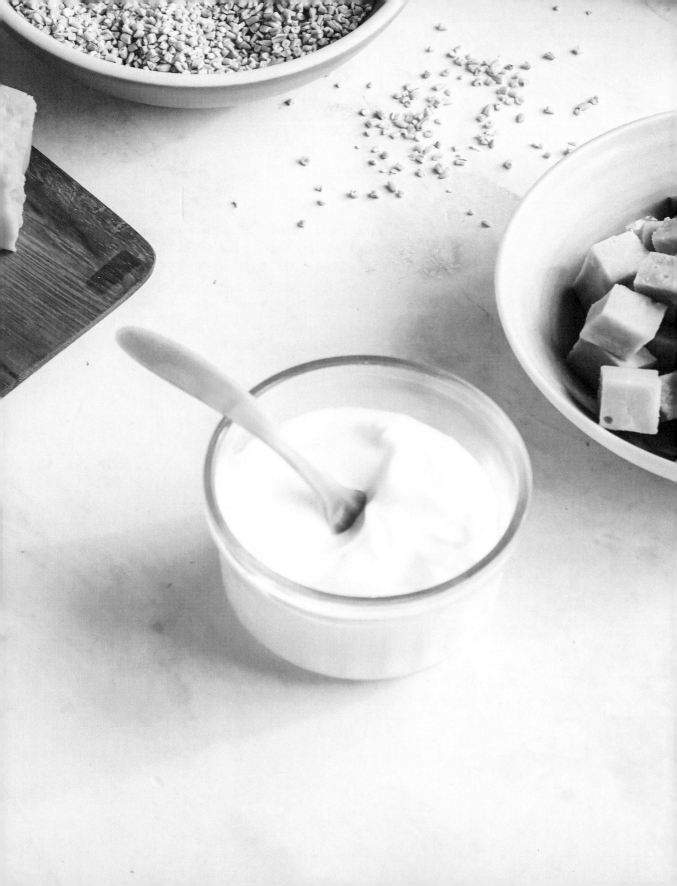

CHAPTER ELEVEN

Dressings, Sauces, and Seasonings

Greek Salad Dressing

MAKES 1 CUP / PREP TIME: 10 MINUTES / TOTAL TIME: 10 MINUTES

When people are trying to lose weight, a lot of effort is put into eating salads. I always get questions about salad dressing. Do I get diet? Or regular? Creamy? Oil-based? Here's the verdict: Diet dressings contain fewer calories, but they are often packed with added sugars and sodium. Oil- and vinegar-based dressings are heart healthy but can still be calorie dense so portions should be limited. There are a lot of options for creamy salad dressings made with yogurt that are suitable replacements for the traditional creamy dressings that are higher in fat. The best dressing? The one you make at home. You can control the ingredients and the flavor is out of this world! The added bonus is you won't ever have to waste time scrutinizing labels in the dressing aisle again.

⅓ cup extra-virgin
   olive oil

Juice of 1 lemon

4 teaspoons minced garlic

1 tablespoon
   dried oregano

1 teaspoon dried basil

½ teaspoon freshly
   ground black pepper

½ teaspoon Dijon
   mustard

½ cup red wine vinegar

Post-Op Servings

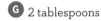 2 tablespoons

1 In a medium bowl, whisk together the olive oil, lemon juice, garlic, oregano, basil, pepper, and mustard. Alternatively, place these ingredients in a dressing shaker bottle and shake until combined.

2 Whisk in the red wine vinegar until emulsified.

3 Serve immediately. Refrigerate any leftovers in an airtight container. When ready to use, let the dressing sit for 10 to 15 minute at room temperature prior to serving in case the oil has solidified. Give it a whisk or a shake before dressing your salad.

Serving tip: *Make salad exciting again by swapping your traditional iceberg lettuce salad for a Mediterranean-inspired Greek salad. Add flavorful dressing to romaine lettuce, sliced red onion, Kalamata olives, pepperoncini, feta cheese, and grilled chicken.*

Per Serving (2 tablespoons): Calories: 89; Total fat: 9g; Protein: 0g; Carbs: 1g; Fiber: 0g; Sugar: 0g; Sodium: 3mg

Creamy Peppercorn Ranch Dressing

MAKES 1 CUP / PREP TIME: 10 MINUTES / TOTAL TIME: 10 MINUTES

For many people ranch dressing is one they can't live without. It not just the most commonly used salad dressing on veggies, but it's also good on burgers, as a dip for almost anything, and as a sandwich spread instead of mayo. The problem with most ranch dressings is that they are loaded with fat, salt, artificial additives, and preservatives. Swap the mayo and heavy cream for Greek yogurt and add natural spices and herbs, toss in a blender, and voilà!— you have a delicious homemade creamy dressing that is the perfect topping for all your favorites.

¾ cup low-fat plain Greek yogurt

⅓ cup grated Parmigiano-Reggiano cheese

¼ cup low-fat buttermilk (see page 76 for tip to make from scratch)

Juice of 1 lemon

2 teaspoons freshly ground black pepper

½ teaspoon onion flakes

¼ teaspoon salt

Post-Op Servings

2 tablespoons

1 In a blender or food processor, puree the yogurt, cheese, buttermilk, lemon juice, pepper, onion flakes, and salt on medium-high speed until the dressing is completely smooth and creamy.

Serving tip: *This ranch dressing is great as a dip for raw vegetables, a condiment for a turkey wrap with vegetables, or a topping for your next turkey burger.*

Per Serving (2 tablespoons): Calories: 35; Total fat: 1g; Protein: 4g; Carbs: 2g; Fiber: 0g; Sugar: 1g; Sodium: 133mg

Seafood Sauce

MAKES 2 CUPS / PREP TIME: 10 MINUTES / TOTAL TIME: 10 MINUTES

We already know that boiled or baked seafood is one of the lowest-calorie ways to eat protein, plus you get all those brain- and heart-healthy omega-3s. But you don't have to eat them plain. Adding a little seafood sauce, rich with flavor from fresh lemon and horseradish, can take your seafood from boring to a zesty party in your mouth.

1½ cups catsup (free of high-fructose corn syrup)

2 tablespoons grated horseradish

Juice of 1 lemon

1 tablespoon Worcestershire sauce

1 teaspoon chili powder

¼ teaspoon freshly ground black pepper

Post-Op Servings

¼ cup

1 In a small bowl, combine the catsup, horseradish, lemon juice, Worcestershire sauce, chili powder, and pepper. Refrigerate, covered, for at least 30 minutes or overnight to let the flavors meld.

2 Serve with shrimp cocktail, oysters, grilled scallops, or other seafood.

Post-op tip: *Use this as a base to enjoy your favorite seafood selections on the pureed diet.*

Per Serving (¼ cup): Calories: 56; Total fat: 0g; Protein: 0g; Carbs: 14g; Fiber: 0g; Sugar: 10g; Sodium: 445mg

Homemade Enchilada Sauce

MAKES 2 CUPS / PREP TIME: 5 MINUTES / COOK TIME: 10 MINUTES
TOTAL TIME: 15 MINUTES

Does this sound familiar? You have all the ingredients to make enchiladas, but you have no sauce. No need to run to the grocery store at the last minute when you can whip up this quick version from simple pantry staples. Mixing all the herbs and seasonings together in a fresh batch makes this sauce super tasty without any added sodium or other artificial ingredients. You might never waste your money on the canned version again!

2 tablespoons extra-virgin olive oil

¼ cup chopped onion

1 teaspoon minced garlic

2 tablespoons whole-wheat pastry flour

1 tablespoon chili powder

½ teaspoon dried oregano

½ teaspoon smoked paprika

1 teaspoon ground cumin

1 cup low-sodium vegetable or chicken broth

½ cup water

1 medium tomato, seeded and chopped

Post-Op Servings

2 tablespoons

1 Place a small saucepan on the stove over medium heat. Add the oil, onion, and garlic. Sauté for 1 to 2 minutes, or until tender.

2 Add the flour. Continue stirring until the onion and garlic are evenly coated.

3 Mix in the chili powder, oregano, paprika, and cumin. Gradually whisk in the broth and water, whisking constantly to prevent lumps from forming.

4 Add the tomato. Cook for 8 to 10 minutes, stirring frequently, or until mixture has thickened. Use an immersion blender to puree the tomato chunks until smooth. Alternatively, transfer the sauce to a blender and puree until smooth.

5 Serve immediately or refrigerate in an airtight container for up to 1 week. You can also freeze and use at a later date.

Per Serving (2 tablespoons): Calories: 37; Total fat: 0g; Protein: 0g; Carbs: 7g; Fiber: 2g; Sugar: 4g; Sodium: 17mg

Mango Salsa

MAKES 2 CUPS / PREP TIME: 15 MINUTES / TOTAL TIME: 15 MINUTES

You can't go wrong using salsa as a condiment. Since it's loaded with simple ingredients, like fresh fruits and vegetables, along with seasonings, it's low in calories and packed with flavor. Just be cautious of what you use to dip in the salsa! Try using it more as a sauce and less as a dip for chips. The flavors from the fresh ingredients surpass any jarred version on store shelves. Try this mango salsa over fish, chicken, crab cakes, or on tacos.

1 large mango, peeled and diced

¼ cup fresh cilantro, finely chopped

Juice of 2 limes

1 jalapeño pepper, stemmed, seeded, and diced

¼ large red onion, finely diced (about ¼ cup)

1 In a medium bowl, mix together the mango, cilantro, lime juice, jalapeño, and onion.

2 Enjoy immediately or refrigerate in an airtight container for up to 3 days.

Per Serving (¼ cup): Calories: 27; Total fat: 0g; Protein: 0g; Carbs: 7g; Fiber: 1g; Sugar: 6g; Sodium: 1mg

Post-Op Servings

¼ cup

Perfect Basil Pesto

MAKES 5 TABLESPOONS / PREP TIME: 5 MINUTES / TOTAL TIME: 5 MINUTES

Pesto isn't just for pasta. It's also an easy-to-make flavorful spread for meat and burgers, or a tasty topping for zoodles. It's also a great way to use up the overabundance of basil in your summer garden. Remember to think of pesto as a fat, not a sauce. You need to use only a very small amount to get loads of flavor in your food. Divide it into mini containers and freeze. Then you just need to thaw one small portion at a time.

1 cup fresh basil leaves

¼ cup Parmigiano-Reggiano cheese

2½ tablespoons extra-virgin olive oil

2 tablespoons pine nuts

2 tablespoons water

Post-Op Servings

1 tablespoon

1 Place the basil, Parmigiano-Reggiano, olive oil, pine nuts, and water in a food processor or blender. Pulse until smooth.

2 Serve immediately or keep in an airtight container before serving.

Ingredient tip: *Pine nuts can be pricey. You may substitute an equal portion of walnuts or almonds as a quick and inexpensive replacement for pine nuts.*

Per Serving (1 tablespoon): Calories: 99; Total fat: 10g; Protein: 2g; Carbs: 1g; Fiber: 0g; Sugar: 0g; Sodium: 68mg

Marinara Sauce with Italian Herbs

MAKES 3 CUPS / PREP TIME: 5 MINUTES / COOK TIME: 35 MINUTES
TOTAL TIME: 40 MINUTES

Marinara is a versatile sauce that can be used to top chicken breasts, tossed with ground meat and beans for a quick chili, or used as a dip for Baked Zucchini Fries (page 79)! Many of the jarred marinara sauces on store shelves are packed with added sugar and salt. Make this quick homemade version. It is full of flavor, and it is rich in the phytochemical lycopene, which protects against cancer.

1 teaspoon extra-virgin olive oil

2 teaspoons minced garlic

½ large yellow onion, finely diced

1 medium red bell pepper, washed, seeded, and finely diced

10 to 12 fresh whole tomatoes, chopped, or 1 (28-ounce) can crushed tomatoes

1 teaspoon dried oregano

¼ teaspoon red pepper flakes

1 teaspoon dried basil

2 bay leaves

1 Place a saucepan over medium heat.

2 Heat the olive oil and garlic for 1 minute.

3 Add the onion and red bell pepper. Cook for 1 to 2 minutes, stirring frequently, or until tender.

4 Add the tomatoes, oregano, red pepper flakes, and basil. Gently stir to combine.

5 Add the bay leaves.

6 Cover, reduce the heat to medium-low, and let simmer for 30 minutes.

Post-Op Servings

 2 to 4 tablespoons

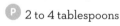

4 tablespoons

7 Remove the cover and discard the bay leaves.

8 Use an immersion blender to puree the marinara to your desired consistency. Alternatively, transfer the sauce to a blender and pulse to achieve your preferred consistency.

Post-op tip: *Use this marinara as a flavorful condiment during the pureed diet to jazz up bland foods. Puree with ground meat, or mix with ricotta or cottage cheese.*

Per Serving (4 tablespoons): Calories: 37; Total fat: 0g; Protein: 0g; Carbs: 7g; Fiber: 2g; Sugar: 4g; Sodium: 17mg

Tips for Eating Out

Wouldn't it be nice if we could have home-cooked meals every single night with clean, fresh ingredients? Although this is a goal, and hopefully something that you have integrated into your lifestyle, there are undoubtedly going to be times when you eat in a restaurant or in someone else's home. Wait until 8 to 12 weeks after surgery before you venture into dining away from home, if at all possible—you will have much better insight about what foods you can tolerate and which ones upset your new stomach.

Here are a few tips to help you follow your weight-loss plan when you are out and about.

▶ **Ask for what you need.** Don't forget, you are paying for the meal and the service when you go out to eat. Ask your server as many questions as needed to make sure you know exactly how your meal is prepared. Let them know you are on a special diet. Some hospitals will provide patients with a special card to hand to the server to make it more discreet.

Boiled, broiled, steamed, poached, and grilled foods are safe bets, and ask twice about sauces. Fried foods are off limits. Period. Make sure you verify that extra butter or oil is not put on your proteins during or after cooking. We know that eating moist food post-op is best tolerated, but in a restaurant most sauces are either high in fat (look for words like *cream, Alfredo, scampi, hollandaise*) or high in sugar (*sweet-and-sour, hoisin*) and should be avoided to prevent illness or taking in extra calories. Broth-based sauces and marinara sauces are the safest bets.

▶ **Investigate ahead of time.** Before you dine out or eat at another person's home, get the menu ahead of time. Most restaurants make their menus available online. That way you'll know how to make a good choice upon arrival, or you can prepare a meal and eat before you go.

▶ **Order à la carte or bring something you can safely eat.** It is likely you won't be able to eat more than a few bites of food, so try ordering just a plain chicken breast, shrimp cocktail, baked fish, or individual flatbread pizza with vegetable toppings. When dining at a friend's or family member's house, review your recipe collection (including this book) to find something that's a crowd pleaser and bring it for everyone to enjoy. That way, if you can't dine on the items your host serves, you'll know you have a safe item to fill you up.

▶ **Having good manners doesn't mean you have to overeat.** Order a doggie bag immediately upon getting your food at the restaurant to avoid the server constantly asking if something was wrong with the meal because you didn't eat much—plus, you don't want a huge plate of uneaten food staring you in the face. At a friend or family member's home, ask for a to-go plate if they insist you taste dessert or something else after you're already full. Then you can decide whether to throw it out once you get home, give it to someone else in the family, or eat it later. Being polite doesn't mean you have to stuff yourself with foods you can't eat or that will push you over your calorie limit.

Measurement Conversions

VOLUME EQUIVALENTS (LIQUID)

US Standard	US Standard (Ounces)	Metric (Approximate)
2 tablespoons	1 fl. oz.	30 mL
¼ cup	2 fl. oz.	60 mL
½ cup	4 fl. oz.	120 mL
1 cup	8 fl. oz.	240 mL
1½ cups	12 fl. oz.	355 mL
2 cups or 1 pint	16 fl. oz.	475 mL
4 cups or 1 quart	32 fl. oz.	1 L
1 gallon	128 fl. oz.	4L

OVEN TEMPERATURES

Fahrenheit (F)	Celsius (C) (Approximate)
250°F	120°C
300°F	150°C
325°F	165°C
350°F	180°C
375°F	190°C
400°F	200°C
425°F	220°C
450°F	230°C

VOLUME EQUIVALENTS (DRY)

US Standard	Metric
⅛ teaspoon	0.5 mL
¼ teaspoon	1 mL
½ teaspoon	2 mL
¾ teaspoon	4 mL
1 teaspoon	5 mL
1 tablespoon	15 mL
¼ cup	59 mL
⅓ cup	79 mL
½ cup	118 mL
⅔ cup	156 mL
¾ cup	177 mL
1 cup	235 mL
2 cups or 1 pint	475 mL
3 cups	700 mL
4 cups or 1 quart	1 L

WEIGHT EQUIVALENTS

US Standard	Metric (Approximate)
½ ounce	15 g
1 ounce	30 g
2 ounces	60 g
4 ounces	115 g
8 ounces	225 g
12 ounces	340 g
16 ounces or	455 g

Resources

Online Resources/Support Communities

Academy of Nutrition and Dietetics

www.eatright.org

The Academy of Nutrition and Dietetics, the largest organization of food and nutrition professionals in America, is a resource for finding credentialed experts in your area. Additionally, the academy's website is a reference for reliable food and nutrition information grounded in expert research.

Alcoholics Anonymous

www.aa.org

Check out this website for information about joining Alcoholics Anonymous. Type in your zip code to easily find local meeting locations and resources. There is also great information about what to do if you think you may have a drinking problem.

American Society for Metabolic and Bariatric Surgery

www.asmbs.org

The American Society for Metabolic and Bariatric Surgery (ASMBS) is the leading organization in research for improving the treatment of obesity through surgical interventions. ASMBS is a valuable reference for reliable, evidenced-based facts about bariatric surgery and obesity treatment.

Bariatric Pal

www.bariatricpal.com

Founded by a bariatric surgery patient, Bariatric Pal is a social network for staying connected with fellow patients—both pre- and post-operatively—and for other bariatric surgery information. Access free forums and chat rooms specialized for each individual surgery type.

My Fitness Pal–Food and Activity Tracker

www.myfitnesspal.com

People who keep a journal or log of their food intake are more successful with weight loss than those just following a meal plan alone. So use this free food and exercise tracker to monitor food intake and track activity to stay on target with your weight-loss regimen. You can closely monitor individual nutrients, such as protein or sugars. There is also a recipe calculator for determining the nutritional information of your favorite homemade recipes.

Obesity Action Coalition

www.obesityaction.org

Check out the Obesity Action Coalition (OAC) for reliable information about obesity treatment, educational resources, and connecting to local support and advocacy groups. Join the OAC to become a member of this community, which has a strong voice in the movement to both prevent and treat obesity, as well as to fight obesity-related discrimination and weight bias.

ObesityHelp

www.obesityhelp.com

An online support community for individuals and their families who struggle with obesity, ObesityHelp has a variety of resources for connecting with peers through support groups or forums. Forums are categorized based on a variety of topics, including diseases related to obesity and type of bariatric surgery. Additionally, you can find access to a wide variety of educational resources here.

Obesity Society

www.obesity.org

The Obesity Society is an organization dedicated to studying obesity and its treatment. Check out this organization for reliable, up-to-date, evidenced-based information about obesity treatment. Find information here about educational programs and conferences around the country.

References

Academy of Nutrition and Dietetics. "Bariatric Surgery." *Nutrition Care Manual.*
Accessed September 1, 2017. www.nutritioncaremanual.org/about-ncm.

Aills, Linda, Jeanne Blankenship, Cynthia Buffington, Margaret Furtado, and Julie
Parrott. "ASMBS Allied Health Nutritional Guidelines for the Surgical Weight
Loss Patient." *Surgery for Obesity and Related Diseases* 4 (2008): S73–S108.
doi:10.1016/j.soard.2008.03.002.

Centers for Disease Control and Prevention. "Adult Obesity Facts." Accessed
December 1, 2017. www.cdc.gov/obesity/data/adult.html.

Cummings, Sue, and Kellene A. Isom, eds. *Pocket Guide to Bariatric Surgery.* 2nd ed.
Academy of Nutrition and Dietetics, 2015.

Hoyuela, Carlos. "Five-Year Outcomes of Laparoscopic Sleeve Gastrectomy as a
Primary Procedure for Morbid Obesity: A Prospective Study." *World Journal of
Gastrointestinal Surgery* 9.4 (2017): 109-117.

Mechanick, J. I., A. Youdim, D. B. Jones, W. T. Garvey, D. L. Hurley, M. M. McMahon,
L. J. Heinbert, et al. "Clinical Practice Guidelines for the Perioperative, Nutritional,
Metabolic and Nonsurgical Support of the Bariatric Surgery Patient–2013 Update:
Cosponsored by American Association of Clinical Endocrinologists, the Obesity
Society, and American Society for Metabolic & Bariatric Surgery." *Obesity* 21,
no. S1 (March 2013): S1–S27. doi: 0.1002/oby.20461.

Mechanick, J. I., R. F. Kushner, H. J. Surgerman, J. M. Gonzalex-Campoy, M. L.
Collazo-Clavell, A. F. Spitz, C. M. Apovian, et al. "American Association of Clinical
Endocrinologists, the Obesity Society, and American Society for Metabolic and
Bariatric Surgery Medical Guidelines for Clinical Practice for the Perioperative
Nutritional, Metabolic, and Nonsurgical Support of the Bariatric Surgery Patient."
Obesity 17, no. S1 (April 2009): S3–S72. doi:10.1038/oby.2009.28.

Neff, Kristin. "Self-Compassion." Accessed January 2, 2018. self-compassion.org

Recipe Index

Index

Acknowledgments

Thank you to my husband, fellow chef, and best friend, Christopher, for supporting all of my adventures as a dietitian. If I could pick one person in the entire world to share a meal with, it would be you.

To E and L. Thank you for giving me a whole new adventure in cooking and eating with each of you. You continue to make dinner time—family time—my favorite part of the day.

To my family. Each and every one of you has inspired at least one of the recipes in this book with your talented culinary skills. Thank you for all the memories shared together over home-cooked meals.

To each and every client and patient I have met with over the years. Thank you for sharing your journey with me. Your smiles, laughs, tears, joys, and frustrations have inspired me in more ways than one to become a better dietitian. Remember never to give up on your journey to be the best you.

Many of the recipes in this book, cooking techniques and tips have been inspired by dozens of fellow dietitians (especially Amy, Joelle, Michelle, Stephanie) and co-workers at Froedtert Health. Thank you for your guidance over the years and mutual love of food. I have learned so much from all of you!

To my lifelong friends—JACKKS. Thank you for always providing a listening ear, love, and support. You have encouraged me to diversify my palate and experiment with meals and cooking.

This book would not have been possible without the support of the comprehensive weight-loss team and bariatric surgery program at Froedtert Health—especially Keri. Each and every one of the nurses, surgeons, providers, and administrative staff helped me learn about how to create a better experience for the patients undergoing bariatric surgery and help them achieve long-term weight-loss success.

Finally, to Stacy Wagner-Kinnear and the editorial, design, and production teams at Callisto Media who provided the opportunity to publish a second book and assisted in all the amazing final finishes to make this cookbook complete. Thank you for your incredibly talented team of creative and hardworking professionals.

About the Author

Sarah Kent, MS, RDN, CSOWM, CD, is passionate about helping people overcome the barriers that prevent them from achieving their nutrition and weight-loss goals. She is the author of the bestselling *Fresh Start Bariatric Cookbook*. For seven years, she served as lead dietitian for the bariatric surgery program at Froedtert & the Medical College of Wisconsin, a nationally certified Center of Excellence for bariatric surgery. She offered a range of nutritional services to both pre- and post-operative bariatric patients and helped facilitate support groups. A registered dietitian nutritionist with a master's degree in human nutrition, Sarah also is a certified specialist in obesity and weight management through the Academy of Nutrition and Dietetics. Sarah, her husband Chris, their two children, and their dog Ladis, live in a suburb of Milwaukee, Wisconsin.